**Neurodegenerative Diseases –
Laboratory and Clinical Research Series**

# SPASTICITY AND ITS MANAGEMENT WITH PHYSICAL THERAPY APPLICATIONS WITH MULTIPLE SCLEROSIS PATIENTS

# NEURODEGENERATIVE DISEASES – LABORATORY AND CLINICAL RESEARCH SERIES

**Multidisciplinary Management of Amyotrophic Lateral Sclerosis**
*J.A. Rocha and D.A. McKim*
2009. ISBN: 978-1-60741-062-1

**Progress in Neurodegeneration: The Role of Metals**
*Maria Rosa Avila-Costa and Veronica Anaya Martinez (Editors)*
2009. ISBN: 978-1-60741-317-2

**Spasticity and its Management with Physical Therapy Applications with Multiple Sclerosis Patients**
*Kadriye Armutlu (Editor)*
2010. ISBN: 978-1-60876-184-5

Neurodegenerative Diseases –
Laboratory and Clinical Research Series

# SPASTICITY AND ITS MANAGEMENT WITH PHYSICAL THERAPY APPLICATIONS WITH MULTIPLE SCLEROSIS PATIENTS

## KADRIYE ARMUTLU
### EDITOR

Nova Science Publishers, Inc.
*New York*

LIBRARY OF CONGRESS CATALOGING-IN-PUBLICATION DATA

Armutlu, Kadriye.
  Spasticity and its management with physical therapy applications / Kadriye Armutlu, Ayla Fil, and Yeliz Özçelik.
    p. ; cm.
  Includes bibliographical references and index.
  ISBN 978-1-60876-184-5 (softcover)
  1. Spasticity--Physical therapy. I. Fil, Ayla. II. Özçelik, Yeliz. III. Title.
  [DNLM: 1. Muscle Spasticity--therapy. 2. Multiple Sclerosis--physiopathology. 3. Multiple Sclerosis--therapy. 4. Physical Therapy Modalities. WE 550 A739s 2009]
  RC935.S64A76 2009
  616.89'13--dc22
                            2009036307

*Published by Nova Science Publishers, Inc. ✛ New York*

# CONTENTS

# Contents

# FOREWORD

There has been an extensive escalation of information on the immunopathogenesis, diagnosis, imaging and therapy of multiple sclerosis in the past 20 years. MS is a complex disease, and its cure depends upon understanding numerous variables. However, we still have so many ways to go as some of these variables still remain unidentified.

During these recent ten years MS, management, including both pharmacological therapy and physical therapy rehabilitation has been improved, changing positively the natural history of this debilitating disease. MS is a multifactorial and heterogeneous disease, so there are responders and non-responders of these effective approaches; however, in both pharmacological treatment and rehabilitation it is evident that early treatment is more effective. Physical therapy and rehabilitation has always been the complementary side of MS treatments. When effective pharmacological treatments have limited efficacy saving motion and coordination is still your ultimate goal rehabilitation is the balancing side of therapy.

Academic physical therapist Kadriye Armutlu has spent dedicatedly more than 15 years finding effective ways to help MS patients to have better quality of life by means of physical therapy rehabilitation approaches.

In this book, with the experience of being our Neurology Clinic Chief Physical Therapist for more than 15 years and caring for our MS Clinic patients, she is bringing us the comprehensive effective treatment approaches in MS Rehabilitation.

The very difficult management aspects of spasticity, postural mechanics of MS and day to day rehabilitation principles are briefly discussed.

This book is an other message of optimism.

*Rana Karabudak MD. Prof.*
*Hacettepe University,*
*Neurology Department,*
*Chief of Neuroimmunology Unit*

# PREFACE

In the current situation, there are not enough information sources available related to neurological physical therapy and rehabilitation, which is a lack for the physiotherapists who work in this area. This absence of information becomes more obvious when the physical therapy techniques of MS and related spasticity are considered.

This book aims to improve the physiotherapists' knowledge and skills related to management of spasticity in MS patients within the holistic therapy principles. Lots of physical therapy techniques used for the management of spasticity in MS are covered from every aspect in this book. It was aimed to give information to the reader especially about the selection strategies of different evaluation techniques, analyzing skills, and setting up treatment plans that fit to patients' expectations.

This book came to existence as a result of years of experience in the both clinical and academic field of neurological physical therapy and rehabilitation. Therefore, first of all, I want to thank my MS patients and the Ankara Branch of the Multiple Sclerosis Association for believing in me and supporting me in gaining the clinical experience through years.

My special thanks go to my assistants, Specialized Physiotherapist Ayla Fil and Physiotherapist Yeliz Özçelik, for their every kind of support, to Nazli Gelincik Tegin and to Nihan Bulut Born, who is a student of the International Physiotherapy Programme at the Hanze Hogeschool of Groningen for not hesitating to give her help in language corrections.

I also owe my thanks to my friend Physiotherapist Samiye Ata and her husband Yalcin Ata for their limitless support to me.

My biggest thanks to my mother and grandmother for helping me grow up and supporting me with their endless love in every occasion.

Kadriye Armutlu
Ankara  2009

In: Spasticity and Its Management …
Editor: Kadriye Armutlu

ISBN: 978-1-60876-185-5
© 2010 Nova Science Publishers, Inc.

*Chapter 1*

# INTRODUCTION

## *Kadriye Armutlu**

Hacettepe University, Faculty of Health Sciences, Department of Physical
Therapy and Rehabilitation, Neurological Rehabilitation Unit
06100/Ankara/TURKEY

In long-term and progressive neurological diseases, such as multiple sclerosis
(MS) in particular, diagnosis, signs and symptoms deriving from the complexity
of human nervous system, are numerous, which leads to difficulties in diagnostic
and evaluation process for physiotherapists practicing neurological rehabilitation
[1]. Difficulties in achieving standardization leads to a lack of controlled, clinical
evidence oriented studies covering large number of subjects; which is a frustrating
factor in the development of new input data and techniques for the
physiotherapists. [2]. In recent years, there have been an increased number of
publications in this field. However, such publications are focused more on stroke
and emphasize general application methods rather than the management of a
single symptom. On the other hand, spasticity, as a symptom of neurological
diseases is difficult to manage and should be handled individually, demanding an
all-day long encounter.

Although there are quite a number of physiotherapy applications developed
specifically for the management of spasticity, which requires a multidisciplinary
approach in the most extensive sense, and to reduce its effects, the most
fundamental weapons of the physiotherapists are therapeutic exercises. An
experienced physiotherapist is able to minimalize effects of spasticity merely by

---

* Email: karmutlu@hacettepe.edu.tr

use of conventional exercises involving passive, active-assisted and active exercises or by neurophysiology oriented exercises such as the Bobath approach. Success firstly depends on the physiotherapist's knowledge of biomechanics, kinesiology, neuroanatomy, neurophysiology and the ability to review the effects of spasticity in accordance with the above mentioned knowledge, and secondly on matching the findings towards functional goals.

Most MS patients do not consult the physical therapist for only one specific complaint, such as spasticity. Usually, the picture is much more complicated than that. Such complex cases can be overcome by the problem-solving ability of the therapist. Therefore, the ability of solving problems has been described as an integral part of physiotherapy practice [3, 4, 5].

Although spasticity is an MS symptom of major importance, other symptoms and their interactions with spasticity should be evaluated as well as a whole within a holistic treatment principle. Complementary treatment programmes should be patient centered, and planned as a long term therapy and supported by home-exercise programmes. The physiotherapist, when considered as a problem-solver, should be able to enhance the efficacy of treatment programme by determining the methods to avert problems and developing the strategies that provide patient's participation in the programme [6, 7]. In most rehabilitation programmes, lack of patient's active participation is a common problem leading to deficiency of the process. The physical therapist has, thereby, an important role in including the patient actively in the therapy.

This book is designed for the physiotherapists practicing neurological rehabilitation, particularly with MS patients. The main goal is providing information about the basic findings and symptoms of MS and the medical treatment approaches to define spasticity together with its composing mechanisms. In addition to that, the effects of the medical treatment approaches, measurement methods of spasticity, mechanical and neurophysiological basis of physical therapy applications that are developed for this purpose and their effect mechanisms are covered, from a physiotherapist's point of view.

This book consist of the findings of 22 years of clinical physiotherapy and 17 years of MS physical therapy experiences of the writer; harmonized with related findings in general literature, surveyed and collected by two assistants of hers; one working on her doctorate and the other for her Master's degree. The information provided in the book is supported by case stories on a problem-solving basis in order to enlighten the reader throughout the practice of applications.

# REFERENCES

[1]   Porter, S. & Chambers, A. & Smith. C. (2003) *Tidy's Physiotherapy* (edit 13) Butterworth and Heinemann, Edinburg.

[2]   Thompson, A.J. (2000). The effectiveness of neurological rehabilitation in multiple sclerosis. *J Rehabil Res Dev,* 37(4):455-61.

[3]   Newman, H.J. (1985). Identifying problems in clinical problem-solving. Perceptions and interventions with nonproblem-solving behaviors. *Physical Ther* 65 (7):1071-1074.

[4]   Weed, L.L. & Zimny, N.J. (1989). The problem-orientated system, problem knowledge coupling and clinical decision-making. *Physical Ther* 69 (7):565-568.

[5]   Edwards, S. (1996). Neurological Physiotherapy. (edition 1). Churchill Livingstone, New York.

[6]   Kuipers, P. & Foste, M. & Smith, S. & Fleming, J. (2009). Using ICF-Environment factors to enhance the continuum of outpatient ABI rehabilitation: an exploratory study. *Disabil Rehabil,* 31(2):144-51.

[7]   Paltamaa, J. & Sarasoja, T. & Leskinen, E. & Wikström, J. & Mälkiä, E. (2008). Measuring deterioration in international classification of functioning domains of people with multiple sclerosis who are ambulatory. *Phys Ther* 88(2):176-90.

In: Spasticity and Its Management ...        ISBN: 978-1-60876-185-5
Editor: Kadriye Armutlu        © 2010 Nova Science Publishers, Inc.

*Chapter 2*

# OVERVIEW OF MS

## *Kadriye Armutlu**

Hacettepe University, Faculty of Health Sciences, Department of Physical
Therapy and Rehabilitation, Neurological Rehabilitation Unit
06100/Ankara/TURKEY

## 2.1. ABSTRACT

MS is an immune-mediated disease of the central nervous system (CNS)
characterized by inflammatory demyelinating process and axonal loss. It is
more common in women than in men and affects young adults. MS is
analyzed within two basic subcategories these are Relapsing-remitting MS
(RRMS) and Progressive MS.

MRI and computed tomography evoked potential studies, and
cerebrospinal fluid analysis generally is used to diagnose in MS alongside
with clinical findings and neurological examination.

There are a lot of common MS symptoms and signs. But weakness,
fatigue, ataxia, balance deficits, bladder and bowel dysfunctions are more
related to spasticity. With the aim of medical management of MS, different
pharmacological treatment options can be used. Although medicines have
positive effects on MS symptoms and spasticity in particular, they also have
many side effects. These side effects may be affect physical therapy
applications.

---

* Email: karmutlu@hacettepe.edu.tr

Physical therapists must be aware of progression, symptom and types of MS, medicine that is used to treatment MS and medicine's side effects for successful management of MS.

Key words: Multiple sclerosis, demyelinization, incidence, types of multiple sclerosis, physical therapy.

## 2.2. INTRODUCTION

MS is an immune-mediated disease of the central nervous system (CNS) characterized by an inflammatory demyelinating process and axonal loss [1, 2]. Generally, it affects young adults. It is reported that the disease is mostly seen in the age range of 15 to 50, with the average diagnostic age being 30. Regarding the population, it is known that the disease is 2:1 more common in women than in men. MS also has geographical aspects: it is seen less frequently near the Equator and more prevalent at the north of the Equator. Southern regions are in the low-risk group. MS is more common among the yellow (Asiatic) and white race; the rate is low among the black race and Eskimos. The prevalence of the disease is 150/100.000 in the North United States and 50/100.000 in the South United States [3, 4, 5].

MS occurs in early years of human life and has a progressive characteristic. The approximate life span of a patient is 40 years after the disease is diagnosed. This period is challenging physically and socially because of the disabilities caused by MS. Within the first 15 years following the diagnosis, about 50% of the patients grow dependent on walkers and 29% on wheelchairs in order to ambulate [6]. Socioeconomical problems related to the disease are huge as well. Direct and indirect cost of the disease to the patient within ten years is approximately $50.000 to $62.000 [7, 8].

MS symptoms, its activation, disability and impairment caused by the disease are dependent on various factors. Symptoms may vary depending on the localization of plaques and demyelinization degree. MS plaques are mostly located in optical nerves, periventricular white matter, corpus callosum, brain stem, cerebellum and spinal cord [9, 10]. For instance, consistency of plaques in the cerebellum and brain stem results in ataxia, tremor and cranial nerve symptoms; whereas plaques in the spinal cord cause pyramidal symptoms (loss in muscle strength and spasticity).

Activation of MS occurs as an outcome of a complex process. Over-activity of cytokines and interleukins is regarded as an important factor. High level of MS activation and rapid progression is generally marked by acute number of relapses within the first two years, forefront cerebellar findings, occurrence in reclining years and patients of male gender. Although the disease has a demyelinating character, axonal loss occurs in the background. In specific types of MS and in some patients, axonal loss occurs in the early stages of the disease [11, 12]. However, usually axonal loss occurs as the disease advances. Demyelinization is a recoverable process, whereas axonal loss is not; therefore axonal loss is regarded as **responsible for the development of patient's disabilities. Studies concerning** MS patients with axonal loss show that such patients have characteristic cerebral atrophies resulting in significant loss in cognitive processes.

## 2.3. MS And PATHOPHYSIOLOGY

MS is a chronic inflammatory demyelinating disease of the central nervous system. The belief that genetic, environmental (infectious agents) and auto-immune factors are effective on the etiology of the disease has become more popular in recent years.

The risk of MS occurrence among individuals whose first-degree relatives are presently suffering or have suffered from the disease is significantly high. Incidence of MS in normal population is 0.1%; whereas the rate is 3% if immediate relatives have MS, and the rate is as high as 25% in twins. According to the findings of recent genome studies IL2R, IL7R and CD58, MS is defined as suspicious alleles as well.

According to the environmental (infectious agents) theory, Chlamydia pneumoniae, human herpes virus-6 and Epstein-Barr virus are responsible for the development of MS. On the other hand, the viewpoint that the disease is not generated merely from environmental factors has also gained importance [13, 14, 15].

According to the auto-immune theory, MS is generated by the myelin antigen-specific CD4+T cells activated in the peripheral immune system getting through the blood-brain barrier. The blood-brain barrier damage leads to myelin destruction.

There are still ongoing studies concerning these three theories.

# 2.4. TYPES OF MS

MS is analyzed within two basic subcategories by most researchers [2]:

## 2.4.1. Relapsing-Remitting MS (RRMS)

This is the most frequently encountered form of MS that shows itself as unpredictable relapses (attacks) and following recovery periods (remissions). Frequency of attacks varies from one patient to another. Eighty percent of MS population is subject to RRMS. Although the lesion is hyperintense, it doesn't enhance with gadolinium on the MRI and localization of plaques are often limited with cerebrum. Disability does not occur in the early stages of this type of disease, and the accumulation of unrecovered impairments may result in a disability formation as the disease progresses. However, these disabilities may not be severe enough to affect patient's daily activities and quality of life in a significant manner.

## 2.4.2. Progressive MS

In progressive MS, there are no distinct attacks. The symptoms worsen progressively during the course of the disease. It consists mainly three subcategories:

### *Primary progressive MS (PPMS)*
Approximately 15 to 20% of MS population has primary progressive form of MS. The course of the disease is characterized by gradual progression from the beginning, with no distinct relapses. Demyelinization plaques are usually located in the spinal cord and have high inflammatory activity. Disability is severe, and the patients become functionally dependent most of the time.

### *Secondary Progressive MS (SPMS*
Following the five years of initial period of RRMS, about 50% of patients develop secondary progressive MS. Localization of demyelinization plaques shift from cerebrum to spinal cord, brain stem and cerebellum together with the increasing inflammatory activity. From this stage, the existing impairments turn into disabilities. The patient becomes functionally dependent and his quality of life deteriorates [16].

*Progressive Relapsing MS (PRMS)*

It is a rare course of MS affecting 5% of the MS Population. The disease continues to progress without remission periods following the relapses. It results in spinal cord lesions and severe disability.

## 2.5. SYMPTOMS OF MS

Symptoms of MS have a wide range and appear in different combinations in the early and later stages of the disease. Primary symptoms are: optic neuritis resulting directly from demyelinization or axonal loss, spasticity, ataxia, tremor, numbness, weakness, balance deficits and cognitive problems. Secondary symptoms are consequences of the primary symptoms. These are: urinary tract infections developing as a result of bladder problems, weakness, balance deficits, loss of senses, muscle atrophies resulting from spasticity, osteoporosis and pressure ulcers. Psychosocial, social, vocational, personal, sexual problems and marriage issues are the tertiary symptoms developing gradually as the disease becomes chronic.

A detailed review of primary MS symptoms—such as weakness, ataxia, and balance deficits, fatigue and bladder problems directly affects the patient by decreasing the functional level and aggrevating disabilities—is essential for the reader.

### 2.5.1. Weakness

Muscle weakness is a common complaint of MS patients. Weakness is a motor finding resulting from the effects of MS on pyramidal system [17, 18]. Although it generally develops along with spasticity, there are some cases of muscle weakness without the presence of spasticity. Weakness usually starts during the early stages of MS in the lower extremities, effecting especially m. tibialis anterior, evertors, hamstrings and hip flexors. Although it is not a must, upper extremity muscle groups are affected as the disease progresses. These muscle groups can be listed as: shoulder flexors, abductors, external rotators and elbow, wrist and finger extensors. Muscle weakness may result in forms of different clinical findings in MS patients such as monoparesis, paraparesis, parapilegia, triparesis, quadriparesis and hemiparesis.

When pathophysiological mechanisms of weakness are analyzed, it is seen that weakness develops both centrally and peripherally. Primary central mechanisms develop directly from the combination of various factors such as decreased motor unit firing rate, impaired motor unit recruitment and decreased central motor conduction, generated as a result of the affected pyramidal system. Peripheral factors develop as a result of the imbalance in muscle strength caused by constant contraction of the spastic muscles, whereas the constant stretched position of antagonist muscle leads to decreased sensibility in muscle fibers and increased stimulation threshold. As stimulation decreases, antagonist muscle weakens and its weaker stimulation threshold increases, forming a vicious circle. Although there is no solid proof, the mentioned process is assumed to cause changes in the form of weakened cross-bridges in the mechanical structure of the muscle as well as neural structure, resulting from constant stretched position of the muscle.

## 2.5.2. Ataxia and Balance Deficits

Ataxia develops when cerebellum and its connections, caudal cord conduction system of spinal cord and vestibular system are affected. Most distinctive outcomes of ataxia can be listed as balance deficits, incoordination and kinetic tremors [19, 20]. Ataxia is resistant to medication. It is one of the three symptoms of MS that cause severe disabilities. Ataxia can be analyzed in three categories depending on its outcomes, which are cerebellar, vestibular and sensory. Combined signs related to all three types of ataxia may be observed in MS patients.

### Sensory Ataxia

Develops when the spinal cord is affected due to the interruption of proprioceptive data generating from lower extremities. Romberg's sign is positive in patients with sensory ataxia, and patients use their visual senses in order to compensate the sensory loss. Therefore, patients keep their eyes fixed on the ground while walking on wide support surfaces.

### Vestibular Ataxia

Vestibular system is responsible for initializing postural reactions, adjustments and fixation of eyes. In patients with vestibular ataxia, balance deficits in gravity dependent postures are accompanied by vertigo and nystagmus.

*Cerebellar Ataxia*

Cerebellar ataxia develops as a result of the lesions that affect the cerebellum and/or the afferent and efferent connections of the cerebellum.

Vestibulo-cerebellar dysfunction is related to the flocculonodular lobe (flocculus and nodulus) and involves problems regulating balance and controlling eye movements. This presents with postural instability, in which the person tends to separate the feet on standing to gain a wider base and avoid oscillations (especially posterior-anterior ones); instability is, therefore, worsened when standing with the feet together (irrespective of whether the eyes are open or closed: this is a negative Romberg's test).

Spino-cerebellar dysfunction corresponds to the vermis and paravermis and presents with a wide-based "drunken sailor" gait, characterized by uncertain start and stop, lateral deviations, and unequal steps and abnormal inter-joint coordination patterns. When this part of the cerebellum is damaged, gait ataxia or walking in-coordination typically occurs. Cerebro-cerebellar dysfunction indicates a lesion of the deep pontine nuclei connections with the cerebellum, which coordinates planning and monitoring of movements and presents with disturbances in carrying out voluntary, planned movements.

Symptoms associated with cerebellar ataxia include: Dysmetria, tremor, dyssynergia, dysdiadockokinesia, hypotonia, weakness, fatigue and nystagmus. Ataxia when accompanied by spasticity has quite negative effects on walk and mobility in MS patients [21, 22].

## 2.5.3. Fatigue

Fatigue is one of the major symptoms of MS, causing an aggravation in disabilities. According to a study conducted on 656 MS patients, fatigue is reported as a common problem for 78% of the subjects. All patients complained about a decrease in their physical activities 14% needed to rest frequently and 10% had to quit their jobs due to fatigue [23, 24].

MS-related fatigue differs from other kinds of fatigue caused by medical problems, specifically in the means of being aggravated by high temperatures.

MS-related fatigue is categorized in two main groups: subjective and motor (objective).

According to a consensus reached by numerous researchers, subjective fatigue is defined as a "subjective lack of physical and or mental energy that is perceived by the individual or caregiver to interfere with usual or desired activities." Its measurement and evaluation process is quite complicated. There are various scales designed for this purpose, among which the Severity Scale, Impact Scale and Visual Analog Scale are highly preferred [25].

Motor fatigue, on the other hand, is characterized by gradual development of muscle weakness during muscular activity. There are a number of scales such as Walking Fatigue Index designed to measure motor fatigue focusing on performance deteriorations generated during sustained muscle activity [26].

Effects of both subjective and objective fatigue symptoms are fundamental for the physiotherapist to determine appropriate physical therapy programmes and antispastic application methods.

## 2.5.4. Bladder and Bowel Dysfunctions

Ninety-six percent of MS patients encounter bladder problems during the first ten years following the diagnosis. When the connection between spinal cord and brain is interrupted, the control of reflex urinating centre over urethral sphincters is damaged, leading to bladder dysfunctions. Bladder symptoms may be one of the different characteristics depending on the localization of the anatomical lesion. The most frequently encountered MS-related bladder symptoms are frequency, urgency, urge incontinence hesitancy [27, 28].

Most patients suffer from overactive (spastic) bladder, which causes problems in urinary storage. Hypoactive (flaccid) bladder, on the other hand, is characterized by a large, areflexic bladder containing excessive amounts of urine. Both two bladder types cause similar symptoms such as frequency, urgency, urge incontinence and nocturia. Another form of bladder problems is detrusor-sphincter dyssynnergia, which causes hesitancy resulting in an increase in residual urine. In such cases, urine should be evacuated through catheterization. If catheterization is not applied, urinary tract infections generate. In addition, hygiene is of major importance during self-catheterization, which may be infectious itself. Due to painful impulses created by the infection and bladder dilation, spasticity along with other MS symptoms may aggravate. In such cases, the physiotherapist should cooperate with the related specialists.

Physiotherapists practicing MS rehabilitation should be well aware of all the symptoms since the interaction of spasticity with other symptoms may result in various outcomes. All possible symptoms of MS are outlined for a better understanding, in Table 1 below.

**Table 1. Common symptoms and signs of MS**

| Motor Symptoms | Visual Symptoms | Cognitive and |
|---|---|---|
| *Weakness* | *Decreased acuity* | Emotional Symptoms |
| *Spasticity* | *Double vision* | *Depression* |
| *Fatigue* | Bladder/Bowel | *Lability* |
| *Balance deficits* | Symptom | *Memory disturbance* |
| *Cerebellar symptoms* | *Urgency* | *Decreased attention and* |
| *Bulbar symptoms* | *Frequency* | *concentration* |
| *Pathological reflexes* | *Incontinence* | Language symptoms |
| Sensory Symptoms | *Urinary retention* | *Dysartria* |
| *Numbness* | *Constipation* | *Dysphasia* |
| *Pain* | *Sexual Symptoms* | |
| *Paresthesia* | *Impotence* | Others |
| *Dysesthesia* | *Loss of genital sensation* | *Paroxismal syndromes* |
| *Proprioceptive loss* | | *Heat intolerance* |
| *L'Hermitte sign* | | |

# 2.6. DIAGNOSIS FOR MS

MS is diagnosed through clinical findings and neurological examination. There are numerous devices designed to assist the physician during the diagnostic process. Such as;

- MRI and computed tomography (used to verify the existence of demyelinization plaques, their density and localization) (figures 1 and 2)
- Evoked potential studies (motor, somatosensory, brain stem auditory and visual)
- cerebrospinal fluid analysis (increase in gamma globulin level and detection of white blood cells)

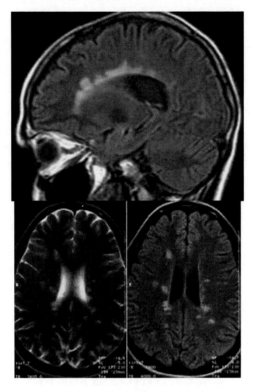

Figure 12: MRI images of MS plaques in periventricular white matter and corpus callosum

In order to provide further assistance to the physician, Poser developed certain criteria in 1984. These guidelines, called Poser Criteria, are as follows [29]:

**Poser Criteria**

*Definite MS*
Two attacks and clinical evidence of two separate lesions
Two attacks, clinical evidence of one and laboratory
evidence of another separate lesion

*Probable MS*
Two attacks and clinical evidence of one lesion
One attack and clinical evidence of two lesions
One attack, clinical evidence of one lesion, laboratory
evidence for another separate lesion

As a member of the rehabilitation team, a well-defined diagnosis is important for the physiotherapist in order to determine his treatment goals. Patients who are diagnosed with MS should be monitored more closely and frequently by the physiotherapist. On the other hand, in cases of probable MS, since the disease is not activated yet, the follow-up examination of the patient may be less frequent.

## 2.7. MEDICAL TREATMENT STRATEGIES AND THEIR EFFECTS ON PHYSICAL THERAPY APPLICATIONS

Medical treatment may be categorized in three groups: immunosuppressive, immunomodulator and others.

Use of steroids is the most common immunosuppressive treatment. Resting and use of steroids form the basis of treatment in cases with acute relapses. Although commonly used, the proper dosage and route of applications are still controversial. Corticosteroids are frequently used as 1gr.of methylprednisolone intravenously for three to five days. Oral intake protocol is started with a total daily dosage of 60 mg, dosage is gradually decreased and discontinued. Some neurologists prefer to use 1gr of methylprednisolone intravenously for a period of one month, prophetically [30].

While application of steroids is effective on RRMS patients, it has minimal or no effect on patients with PPMS, SPMS and RPMS.

Although corticosteroids have positive effects on RRMS symptoms and spasticity in particular, they also have many side effects. These side effects may be defined as acute and chronic. Acute side effects can be listed as tachycardia, perspiration, etc. Chronic side effects can be listed as bone osteoporosis, secondary muscle weakness-atrophy.

**ATTENTION!**
Existence of osteoporosis is crucial for physiotherapy applications and should be taken into consideration while making a prescription for physiotherapy.

Another form of immunosuppressive treatment is the application of low-dosage chemotherapeutic medication. Mitoxantrone, methotrexate, azathioprine, etc. are the most widely used medications [31].

Beta-interferons beta 1b (Betaseron® ve Betaferon®) and 1a (Avonex™ ve Rebif®) are highly preferred during immunomodulation treatments. Both beta 1a and 1b are used for managing the frequency and severity of relapses in the course of RRMS. In recent years, interferon beta 1b is also used for decelerating the progression of disabilities developing along with SPMS [32]. Beta interferons have a wide range of side effects; the ones concerning the physiotherapists are summed up in Table 2.

Plasma exchange is an alternative treatment method for patients who do not respond to the immunosuppressive and immunomodulator treatments and whose disease course has rapid progression. Plasma exchange is applied for five to ten sessions, and during the treatment, physical therapy programme should be recessed in order to enable the patient to rest.

In recent years, newly developed medications are under trial on MS patients. Among these, Rituximab is frequently used by RRMS patients and Natalizumab by SPMS patients [33, 34]. The side-effect profile of such medications not definite yet, therefore, there is no absolute information about their effects on physical therapy applications.

Apart from the mentioned treatments, alternative collateral medications such as statines, estrogen, B12 supplement may be used as well.

**Table 2. Side effects of beta-interferon application and negative effects on the physiotherapy programme**

| Side-effects | Effects |
| --- | --- |
| Flu-like symptoms (lasts for one to two days following the injection) | Physiotherapy programme should be recessed |
| Cutaneous necroses | Increases spasticity and spasms by generating painful stimulants |
| increase in the severity of spasticity permanently | More aggressive methods should be used in order to manage spasticity |
| Inflamed injection sites | Increases spasticity and spasms by generating painful stimulants |

Some diseases have scales of global use, designed for measuring the effects of treatments, monitoring progression and phases of the disease. One of those is Expanded Disability Status Scale (EDSS), used for the assessment of MS, which was developed by Kurtzke and improved by other researchers later on [35] (see appendix 1). By use of this scale, mainly eight functional systems, which can be listed as pyramidal, cerebellar, brain stem, sensory, bladder-bowel, visual, cerebral functions and others, are analyzed. Outcomes are scored from zero to ten, according to mobilization formation and distance.

## 2.8. CONCLUSION

MS is more prevalent among young adults and in women with a ratio of 2:1. It also consists of various symptoms. The disease shows itself in early ages; the patient is detached from work and social life during his most productive years, particularly by reason of problems in mobility. On this account, in the first 15 years following the diagnosis, 50% of MS patients become dependent on walkers and 29% on wheelchairs in order to ambulate. In the first ten years, 50 to 80% of MS patients lose their jobs. This rate constitutes a large number of occupational losses among young adult population.

Primary symptoms of MS are: optic neuritis, spasticity, ataxia, tremor, numbness, weakness, balance deficits and cognitive problems. Secondary symptoms are: urinary tract infections, muscular atrophies, osteoporosis and pressure ulcers. In addition to those, tertiary symptoms are psychosocial, social, vocational, personal, sexual problems and marriage issues.

MS has numerous primary and secondary symptoms; the intensity and severity vary according to MS subtypes as well. For instance, spasticity and loss of strength stand out in PPMS, whereas sensory problems are more frequently encountered in RRMS. Management of spasticity may be actualized by exercising complementary physiotherapy programmes. The physical therapist should focus on the symptoms of major importance, such as weakness, fatigue, ataxia and bladder/bowel problems.

There are quite a large number of pharmacological treatment options developed for the medical management of MS. These medications have specific side effects that may have direct or indirect effects on physical therapy programmes. Long-term use of corticosteroids in particular may result in osteoporosis and use of interferons aggravates the spasticity.

Physiotherapists working in the field of neurology, MS in particular, should have a good knowledge of medical treatment strategies and be aware of pharmalogical side effects related to MS in order to improve the efficiency of the physical treatment programme.

## 2.9. REFERENCES

[1] Compston A, Coles A. Multiple sclerosis (seminar) *Lancet*, 2002;359: 1221-1231.

[2] Schapiro RT. Introduction. *International journal of MS care*, (Suppl). 2006. 4-5.

[3] Orsini JA, Dombovy ML. Multiple sclerosis and Parkinson's disease rehabilitation. Hapter 12. Lazar RB (ed). McGraw-Hill, New York, 173-197, 1998.

[4] Dean G, Kurtzke JF. On the risk of multiple sclerosis according to age at immigration to South Africa. *Br Med J.*, 1971. 3:725.

[5] Confavreux, C. & Vukusic, S. (2008). The clinical epidemiology of multiple sclerosis. *Neuroimaging Clin N Am,* 18(4):589-622.

[6] Confavreux, C. & Vukusic, S.& Moreau, T. (2000 )Adeleine Relapses and progression of disability in multiple sclerosis. *N Engl J Med*, 16;343(20):1430-8.

[7] Brown, T.R. & Kraft, G.H. (2005). Exercise and rehabilitation for individuals with multiple sclerosis. *Phys Med Rehabil Clin N Am,* 16(2):513-55.

[8] Birnbaum H.G. & Ivanova, J.I. & Samuels, S. & Davis, M. & Cremieux, P.Y. & Phillips, A.L. & Meletiche, D. (2009). Economic impact of multiple sclerosis disease-modifying drugs in an employed population: direct and indirect costs. *Curr Med Res Opin,* 25(4):869-77.

[9] Chang, A.& Smith, M.C. & Yin, X. & Fox, R.J. & Staugaitis, S.M. & Trapp, B.D. (2008). Neurogenesis In The Chronic Lesions Of Multiple Sclerosis. *Brain,* 131(9):2366-75.

[10] Stankiewicz, J.M. & Neema, M. & Alsop, D.C. & Healy, B.C. & Arora, A.& Buckle, G.J. & Chitnis, T.& Guttmann, C.R. & Hackney, D. & Bakshi, R. (2009). Spinal cord lesions and clinical status in multiple sclerosis: A 1.5 T and 3 T MRI study. *J Neurol Sci.* 2009 Apr 15; 279(1-2):99-105.

[11] Peterson, J.W. & Bö, L. & Mörk, S. & Chang, A. & Trapp, B.D. (2001). Transected neurites, apoptotic neurons, and reduced inflammation in cortical multiple sclerosis lesions. *Ann Neurol,* 50(3):389-400.

[12] Perry, V.H. & Woolley, S.T. & Anthony, D.C.(1999) The role axonal pathology in MS disability. *The International MS Journal,* 6; (1):7-13.

[13] Gutiérrez, J. & Koppel, B &. Kleiman, A. & Akfirat, G. (2008). Multiple sclerosis and Epstein-Barr virus: a growing association. *Rev Med Inst Mex Seguro Soc,* 46(6):639-42.

[14] Lincoln, J.A. & Hankiewicz, K. & Cook, S.D. (2008). Could Epstein-Barr virus or canine distemper virus cause multiple sclerosis? *Neurol Clin,* 26(3):699-715.

[15] Pugliatti, M. & Harbo, H.F. & Holmøy, T. & Kampman, M.T. & Myhr, K.M. & Riise, T. & Wolfson, C. (2008). Environmental risk factors in multiple sclerosis. *Acta Neurol Scand Suppl,* 188:34-40.

[16] Rovaris, M. & Confavreux, C.& Furlan, R. & Kappos, L. & Comi, G. & Filippi, M. (2006) Secondary progressive multiple sclerosis: current knowledge and future challenges. *Lancet Neurol,* 5(4):343-54.

[17] Reich, D.S. & Zackowski, K.M. & Gordon-Lipkin, E.M. & Smith, S.A. & Chodkowski, B.A. & Cutter, G.R. & Calabresi, P.A. (2008). Corticospinal tract abnormalities are associated with weakness in multiple sclerosis. *AJNR Am J Neuroradio,*29(2):333-9.

[18] Carroll, C.C. & Gallagher, P.M. & Seidle, M.E. & Trappe, S.W. (2005). Skeletal muscle characteristics of people with multiple sclerosis. *Arch Phys Med Rehabil,* Feb;86 (2):224-9.

[19] Schapiro, R.T. (2001). Management of spasticity, pain and paroxysmal phenomena in multiple sclerosis. *Current neuroscience Rep,* 1:299-302.

[20] Gibson-Horn, C. (2008). Balance-based torso-weighting in a patient with ataxia and multiple sclerosis: a case report. *J Neurol Phys Ther,* 32(3):139-46.

[21] Mills, R.J. & Yap, L. & Young, C.A. (2007). Treatment for ataxia in multiple sclerosis. *Cochrane Database Syst Rev,* 24;(1):CD005029.

[22] Brown, T.R. & Kraft, G.H. (2005). Exercise and rehabilitation for individuals with multiple sclerosis. *Phys Med Rehabil Clin N Am,* 16(2):513-55.

[23] Shah, A. (2009). Fatigue in multiple sclerosis. *Phys Med Rehabil Clin N Am,* 20(2):363-72.

[24] Kos, D. & Kerckhofs, E. & Nagels, G. & D'hooghe, M.B. & Ilsbroukx, S. (2008). Origin of fatigue in multiple sclerosis: review of the literature *Neurorehabil Neural Repair,* 22(1):91-100.

[25] MacAllister, W.S. Krupp, L.B. (2005). Multiple sclerosis-related fatigue. *Phys Med Rehabil Clin N Am,* 16(2):483-502.

[26] Schwid, S.R. Covington, M. Segal, B.M. Goodman, A.D. (2002). Fatigue in multiple sclerosis: current understanding and future directions. *J Rehabil Res Dev,* 39(2):211-24.

[27] Nortvedt, M.W. & Riise, T. & Frugård, J. & Mohn, J. & Bakke, A.& Skår, A.B. & Nyland, H. & Glad, S.B. & Myhr, K.M. (2007). Prevalence of bladder, bowel and sexual problems among multiple sclerosis patients two to five years after diagnosis. *Mult Scler,* 13(1):106-12.

[28] De, Ridder D. & Ost, D, Van der Aa, F. & Stagnaro, M. & Beneton, C. & Gross-Paju, K. & Eelen, P. & Limbourg, H. & Harper, M. & Segal, J.C. & Fowler, C.J. & Nordenbo, A. (2005). Conservative bladder management in advanced multiple sclerosis. *Mult Scler,* 11(6):694-9.

[29] Poser, C.M. & Brinar, V.V. (2001). Diagnostic criteria for multiple sclerosis. *Clin Neurol Neurosurg,* 103(1):1-11.

[30] Perumal, J.S. & Caon, C. & Hreha, S.& Zabad, R. & Tselis, A.& Lisak, R.& Khan, O. (2008). Oral prednisone taper following intravenous steroids fails to improve disability or recovery from relapses in multiple sclerosis. *Eur J Neurol,*15(7):677-80.

[31] Pielen, A. & Goffette, S. & Van Pesch, V. & Gille, M. & Sindic, C.J. (2008). Mitoxantrone-related acute leukemia in two MS patients. *Acta Neurol Belg,* 108(3):99-102.

[32] Markowitz, C. (2004). Development of interferon-beta as a therapy for multiple sclerosis. *Expert Opin Emerg Drugs,* 9(2):363-74.

[33] Bourdette, D, & Yadav, V. (2008). B-cell depletion with rituximab in relapsing-remitting multiple sclerosis. *Curr Neurol Neurosci Rep,* 8(5):417-8.

[34] Oturai, A.B. & Koch-Henriksen, & N. Petersen, T. & Jensen, P.E.& Sellebjerg, F. & Sorensen, P.S. (2009). Efficacy of natalizumab in multiple sclerosis patients with high disease activity: a Danish nationwide study. *Eur J Neurol,* 16(3):420-3.

[35] Kurtzke, J.F. (1983). Rating neurologic impairment in multiple sclerosis: an expanded disability status scale (EDSS). *Neurology,* 33(11):1444-52.

# APPENDIX 1

## Functional Systems

The EDSS is based upon Neurological testing of Functional Systems (CNS areas
regulating body functions): Pyramidal (ability to walk), Cerebellar
(Coordination), BrainStem (Speech and Swallowing), Sensory (Touch and Pain),
Bowel and Bladder; Visual; Mental; and "Other" (includes any other
Neurological findings due to Multiple Sclerosis).

Each Functional System (FS) is graded to the nearest possible grade, and V
indicates an unknown abnormality; these are not additive scores and are only
used for comparison of individual items.

**Pyramidal Function**
0 - Normal
1 - Abnormal Signs without Disability
2 - Minimal disability
3 - Mild/Moderate ParaParesis of HemiParesis; Severe MonoParesis
4 - Marked ParaParesis or HemiParesis; Moderate QuadraParesis or
MonoParesis
5 - Paraplegia, Hemiplegia, or Marked ParaParesis
6 - Quadriplegia
V - Unknown

**Cerebellar Function**
0 - Normal
1 - Abnormal Signs without disability
2 - Mild Ataxia
3 - Moderate Truncal or Limb Ataxia
4 - Severe Ataxia
5 - Unable to perform Coordinated Movements
V - Unknown
X - Weakness

**BrainStem Function**
0 - Normal
1 - Signs only
2 - Moderate Nystagmus or other mild disability
3 - Severe Nystagmus, Marked Extra Ocular Weakness or moderate disability of
other Cranial Nerves
4 - Marked Dysarthria or other marked disability

5 - Inability to Speak or <u>Swallow</u>
V - Unknown
**<u>Sensory</u> Function**
0 - Normal
1 - Vibration or Figure - Writing decrease only, in one or two limbs
2 - Mild decrease in Touch or Pain or Position Sense, and/or moderate decrease in Vibration in one or two limbs, or Vibration in three or four limbs
3 - Moderate decrease in Touch or Pain or <u>Proprioception</u>, and/or essentially lost Vibration in one or two limbs; or mild decrease in Touch or Pain and/or moderate decrease in all Proprioceptive tests in three or four limbs
4 - Marked decrease in Touch or Pain or loss of Proprioception, alone or combined in one or two limbs; or moderate decrease in Touch or Pain and/or severe Proprioceptive decrease in more than two limbs
5 - Loss of Sensation in one or two limbs; or moderate decrease in Touch or Pain and/or loss of Proprioception for most of the body below the head
6 - Sensation essentially lost below the head
V - Unknown
**Bowel and <u>Bladder</u> Function**
0 - Normal
1 - Mild Urinary Hesitancy, Urgency, or Retention
2 - Moderate <u>Hesitancy</u>, Urgency, or Retention of Bowel or Bladder, or rare Urinary Incontinence
3 - Frequent Urinary Incontinence
4 - Almost constant Catheterization.
5 - Loss of Bladder function
6 - Loss of Bowel function
V - Unknown
**Visual Function**
0 - Normal
1 - <u>Scotoma</u> with Visual Acuity > 20/30 (corrected)
2 - Worse Eye with Scotoma with maximal Acuity 20/30 to 20/59
3 - Worse Eye with large Scotoma or decrease in fields, Acuity 20/60 to 20/99
4 - Marked decrease in fields, <u>Acuity</u> 20/100 to 20/200; grade 3 plus maximal Acuity of better Eye < 20/60
5 - Worse Eye Acuity < 20/200; grade 4 plus better Eye Acuity < 20/60
V - Unknown
**<u>Cerebral</u> Function**
0 - Normal

1 - <u>Mood alteration</u>
2 - Mild decrease in <u>Mentation</u>
3 - Moderate decrease in Mentation
4 - Marked decrease in Mentation
5 - Dementia
V - Unknown
**Other Function**
0 - Normal
1 - <u>Other Neurological finding</u>


## The Expanded Disability Status Scale (EDSS)

0.0    - Normal Neurological Exam.

1.0    - No disability, minimal signs on one <u>FS</u>.

1.5    - No disability minimal signs on two of seven <u>FS</u>.

2.0    - Minimal disability in one of seven <u>FS</u>.

2.5    - Minimal disability in two <u>FS</u>.

3.0    - Moderate disability in one FS; or mild disability in three to four <u>FS</u>, though fully ambulatory.

3.5    - Fully ambulatory but with moderate disability in one FS and mild disability in  one or two FS; or moderate disability in two FS; or mild disability in five <u>FS</u>.

4.0    - Fully ambulatory without aid, up and about 12hrs a day despite relatively severe disability. Able to walk without aid 500 meters.

4.5    - Fully ambulatory without aid, up and about much of day, able to work a full day, may otherwise have some limitations of full activity or require minimal assistance. Relatively severe disability. Able to walk without aid 300 meters.

5.0    - Ambulatory without aid for about 200 meters. Disability impairs full daily activities.

5.5    - Ambulatory for 100 meters, disability precludes full daily activities.

6.0    - Intermittent or unilateral constant assistance (cane, crutch or brace) required to walk 100 meters with or without resting.

6.5    - Constant bilateral support (cane, crutch or braces) required to walk 20 meters without resting.

7.0    - Unable to walk beyond five meters even with aid, essentially restricted to wheelchair, wheels self, transfers alone; active in wheelchair about 12 hours a day.

7.5    - Unable to take more than a few steps, restricted to wheelchair, may need aid to transfer; wheels self, but may require motorized chair for full day's activities.

8.0    - Essentially restricted to bed, chair, or wheelchair, but may be out of bed much of day; retains self-care functions, generally effective use of arms.

8.5    - Essentially restricted to bed much of day, some effective use of arms, retains some self-care functions.

9.0    - Helpless bed patient, can communicate and eat.

9.5    - Unable to communicate effectively or eat/swallow.

10.0   - Death.

[35] Kurtzke, J.F. (1983). Rating neurologic impairment in multiple sclerosis: an expanded disability status scale (EDSS). *Neurology,*33(11):1444-52.

ISBN: 978-1-60876-185-5
© 2010 Nova Science Publishers, Inc.

*Chapter 3*

# SPASTICITY

## Kadriye Armutlu*

Hacettepe University, Faculty of Health Sciences, Department of Physical
Therapy and Rehabilitation, Neurological Rehabilitation Unit
06100/Ankara/TURKEY

## 3.1. ABSTRACT

Spasticity is an upper motor neuron lesion component caused by the
velocity of exaggerated tendon jerks and muscle tonicity characterized by
excessive tonic reflexes. This typically occurs following multiple sclerosis,
stroke, brain injury (trauma and other causes), spinal cord injury, cerebral
palsy and other disabling neurological diseases. Clasp knife phenomenon and
flexor spasms are associated reactions that accompany spasticity.

Spasticity can be explained by spinal and/or supraspinal mechanisms.
Spinal mechanism of spasticity is still controversial in several ways with its
undetermined aspects. Alterations in motor-neuron inhibition, fusimotor
activity, alterations in the characteristics of motor neurons and morphological
plasticity are considered responsible for the lack of the modulating influence
of supraspinal mechanisms on the spinal cord. Supraspinal mechanism of
spasticity has both similar and dissimilar characteristics with hemiplegic
spasticity, which occurs as an outcome of CVA. Spasticity affects the
antigravity muscles of the body, resulting in hypertonia in the flexor muscles
of upper extremities and extensor muscles of lower extremities. This is an
outcome of rubro-spinal tract, facilitating the motor neurons of upper

---

* Email: karmutlu@hacettepe.edu.tr

extremity flexor muscles and inhibiting the motor neurons of the extensor muscles. Ventromedial reticulospinal tract has a similar effect. Vestibulospinal tract—on the other hand—sends facilitating impulses to the extensory motor neurons of lower body and lower extremity muscles and has inhibitory effects on flexor muscles. Though a similar course may be seen in MS, hypertonia may occur in a more complicated way in unexpected muscle groups. This results from the localization of demyelization plaques.

Keywords: Tonic reflex, hypertonus, multiple sclerosis, spinal mechanism, supraspinal mechanism.

# 3.2. INTRODUCTION

An upper motor neuron lesion develops as a result of damage in the anatomical integrity of the area starting from cerebral cortex to spinal cord's ventral horn motoneurons, caused by hemorrhage, occlusion, demyelinization and trauma (figure 1). This damage is generated in conjuncture with diseases like MS, cerebrovascular accident (CVA) and spinal cord injury (SCI). One of the major signs of upper motor neuron syndrome is spasticity.

In the case of neurological disorders, spasticity is one of the most fundamental symptoms that results in disability. According to the definition made by Lance in 1980, which is still partially valid today, "as a motor disorder, spasticity is an upper motor neuron lesion component caused by the velocity of exaggerated tendon jerks and muscle tonicity characterized by excessive tonic reflexes" [1]. Lance's definition of spasticity includes only the increased velocity dependent stretch reflexes and hyperactive tendon jerks and is thus narrower than some of the clinical uses of the term, but it does have the advantage of being more precise. Some authors have decided to use a more clinically relevant definition, which also includes clonus, spasm and hyperreflexia [2, 3], whereas others have decided to use the more strict definition which focuses on hypertonia [4, 5, 6 ].

Physiotherapists define muscular tonus as "the state of awareness of body segments to actualize a movement or maintain body posture and their ability of adapting to a given movement/position" [7]. Successful voluntary movement requires both a minimal level of this background postural tone and adequate selective muscle activity. Physical therapists use the term spasticity to refer to the collective abnormality in motor control following a UMN lesion. On this account, they prefer to define spasticity as an "impairment of the ability to modulate background tone and loss of selective muscle activation resulting in functional deficit with a state of static fixation, rather than the dynamic stability provided by normal **tone**" [8].

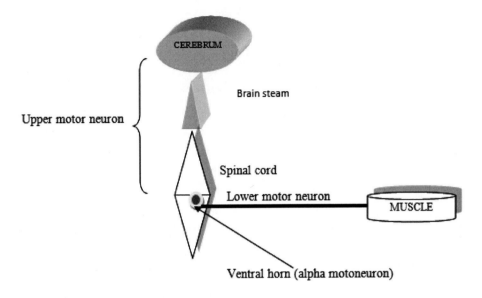

Figure 1. Schematization of upper and lower motor neurons.

In fact, frequently spasticity includes many features of UMN syndrome; however, this may not always be the case [9, 10]. Therefore, an absolute definition of spasticity is not of major importance. It is possible to determine the probable outcomes of spasticity by analyzing the symptoms of UMN syndrome (Table 1).

## 3.3. NEUROPHYSIOLOGY OF SPINAL REFLEXES

This lesion eliminates the effect of supraspinal control system on the spinal cord partially or almost completely, causing alterations in spinal reflex mechanisms resulting in an exaggerated stretch reflex. It will be enlightening for the reader if the stretch reflex and physiologies of neural activities concerning the stretch reflex are reviewed.

Neural circuit of the stretch reflex is formed by the participation of muscle fibers, afferent neurons and sensory neurons (group Ia and group II), inhibitory interneurons located in the intermediate area of the spinal cord and alfa-motor neurons in the ventral horn. Gamma motor neurons, located in the ventral horn of the spinal cord, increase the Ia afferent neuron activity and participate in the tonicity of the muscle by way of contracting poles of muscle fibers through stimulation [11].

**Table 1. Symptoms of upper motor syndrome**

| |
|---|
| **Positive symptoms ( abnormal or exaggerated behaviors )** |
| Enhanced stretch reflexes |
|   Increased muscle tone |
|   Exaggerated tendon reflexes |
|   Clonus |
| Released flexor reflexes |
|   Babinski response |
|   Mass synergy patterns ( i.e., posturing of limbs and trunk certain patterns, such as flexion of upper limb and extension of the lower limb in a stroke patient ) |
| **Negative symptoms ( performance deficits )** |
|   Loss of finger dexterity |
|   Weakness |
|   Loss of selective control of muscles and limb segments |

Muscle fiber is sensitive to muscle length alterations and stretching; it transmits these modifications to medulla spinalis via group Ia and group II afferent neurons. As long as the muscle fibers stretch, group Ia afferents continue to produce impulses in direct proportion with the velocity and intensity of the stretching. This process is called "dynamic response of primary muscle endings." Group II afferents are also stimulated by the stretching of muscle fibers, but they continue to send impulses even after stretching ends. This is called "static response of secondary endings." Muscle fiber has maximal activation when the muscle is in its most stretched position. As the muscle starts to contract, activation of the fiber declines and the fiber's activation diminishes when the muscle reaches maximum contraction (figure 2). Following the synapse of group Ia and group II afferent neurons to the spinal ganglion, they enter the spinal cord through the posterior pedunculus. Both afferents generate a monosynaptic connection with alfa motoneurons, causing the contraction of extrafusal muscle fibers—in other words, providing the formation of stretching reflex. The distinction between the effects of the two afferent groups is that group Ia generates a short latency stretching reflex whereas group II generates a long latency stretching reflex [12].

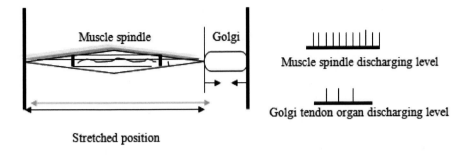

Figure 2. Activation of muscle spindle and golgi tendon organ when the muscle is in stretched position.

Another receptor of the muscle is golgi tendon organ. During the muscle contraction, sensitive to the muscle under tension, golgi tendon organ sensation is transmitted to the spinal cord by group Ib afferent neurons. Ib afferents generate a polysynaptic connection and synapse agonist and antagonist alfa motoneurons. The golgi tendon organ has maximal activation when the muscle reaches maximum contraction. As the muscle relaxes, activation of golgi tendon organ declines (figure 3).

During the formation of stretch reflex, inhibitory interneurons (group Ia, renshaw and others) provide stabilization, or the relaxation of antagonist muscle while agonist muscle contracts, or they halt the agonist action during a voluntary action by stimulating the antagonist muscle and reversing the action. Inhibitory interneurons function by way of postsynaptic inhibition. The first of these inhibitions is reciprocal inhibition (group Ia inhibition). This is required for agonist-synergistic muscle contraction and antagonist muscle relaxation. Inhibition of antagonist muscle is provided by the polysynaptic connection of group Ia afferents with group Ia inhibitory interneurons. Renshaw inhibition (recurrence) occurs when group Ia afferents enter the spinal cord and synapse the nearby renshaw inhibitory interneurons. Through the synapse, renshaw inhibitory interneurons inhibit the alfa motor neurons stimulated by group Ia afferents and halt the agonist movement when required. Furthermore, group Ia afferents inhibit the inhibitory interneurons inhibiting the agonist muscle (disinhibition) and remove the inhibition of antagonist muscle (figure 4).

The function of autogenetic inhibition is presumed to be the protection of the muscle from injuries caused by over-contractions. When the impulses generating from golgi tendon organ are transmitted to the spinal cord through group Ib afferents, golgi bottle neuron synapse inhibitor interneurons, inhibiting the alfa motoneurons of the stimulated muscle and facilitate the alfa motor neurons of antagonist muscle (figure 5). Inhibition of group II generally has facilitating effects on alfa motor neurons of flexor muscles and inhibitory effects on extensor muscles. Controlled by supraspinal centers, spinal reflex activation is modulated properly [13].

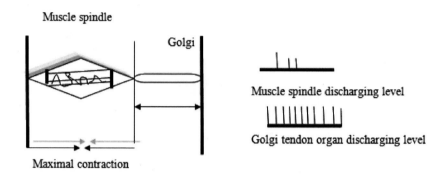

Figure 3. Activation of muscle spindle and golgi tendon organ during maximal contraction.

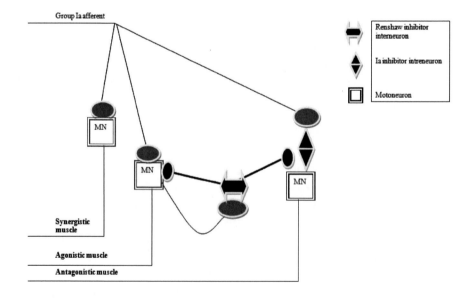

Figure 4. Reciprocal and renshaw inhibitions.

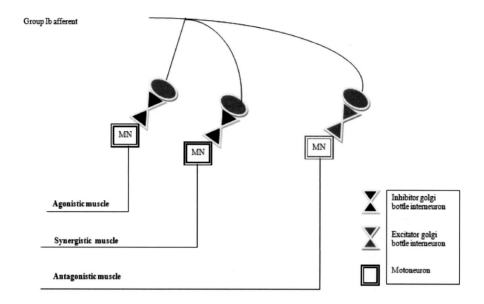

Figure 5. Autogenic inhibition.

## 3.4. SPINAL MECHANISM OF SPASTICITY

Spasticity is an upper motor neuron symptom occurring in spinal and/or supraspinal mechanisms. Spasticity in MS occurs either when supraspinal anatomic areas are affected or when solely the spinal anatomic areas are affected or when both areas are affected due to localization of demyelinization plaques and axonal loss. Axonal losses and plaques located in different parts of the spinal cord result in incomplete cord lesion. Accordingly, differences related to muscle groups affected by spasticity in MS patients are an expected result. Clinically, lateral corticospinal tract and dorsal reticulospinal tract are affected similarly in the case of partial cord lesions. Therefore, spasticity with an effect on the lower extremity antigravity muscles occurs. In rare cases, spasticity may affect the flexor muscles in accordance with the areas affected in the spinal cord.

Spinal mechanism of spasticity is still controversial in several ways with its undetermined aspects. Alterations in motor-neuron inhibition, fusimotor activity and in the characteristics of motor neurons and morphological plasticity are considered responsible for the lack of the modulating influence of supraspinal mechanisms on the spinal cord.

## 3.4.1. Changes in Motor-Neuron Inhibition

During the formation of the voluntary movement, the influence of presynaptic and postsynaptic inhibitions on the spinal motor-neuron activity is important. Hereafter, the influence of three inhibitions becomes pathological and their roles on the spinal mechanisms of spasticity are to be discussed.

### *Alteration of Reciprocal Ia Inhibition*

Disynaptic reciprocal Ia inhibition—a segmental reflex—is believed to decline in spinal spasticity. Studies on the gastrocnemius and tibialis anterior muscles of MS patients show that, due to the declining reciprocal Ia inhibition, tibialis anterior fails to perform the required activation and gastrocnemius is not able to relax [14]. Moreover, uncontrolled Ia inhibitory interneurons caused by descending pathways result in spastic co-contraction [15].

### *Alteration of Recurrent Inhibition*

Recurrent inhibition (renshaw inhibition), which sets in when a voluntary agonist movement requires to be stopped in a healthy person, alters as a result of upper motor lesions leading to uncontrolled pathways. According to some researchers, this alteration is in the direction of an increase, whereas to some others, it is in the direction of a decrease. This controversy results from the complications in evaluating recurrent inhibition in human beings. However, it is clear that modulation of the inhibition is damaged [16, 17, 18, 19]. Damaged modulation of the recurrent inhibition is regarded as a cause of spastic co-contraction by declining the Ia reciprocal inhibition [20].

### *Alteration of Autogenic Inhibition*

Studies show that Ib afferent pathway has both inhibitory and excitatory effects. SCI likely has a crucial role in the pathophysiology of spasticity since it decomposes this inhibitory/excitatory balance.

### *Fusimotor Activity*

Gamma motor neurons are capable of producing spontaneous discharge. Supraspinal centers minimalize this process and solely allow discharges required for the continuity of the muscle tonicity. It was assumed that spinal lesion abated this control mechanism, which resulted in an increase in the stimulation of gamma motor neurons to the muscle fiber poles, decrease in muscle fiber threshold and a resistance to passive movement. However, these presumptions retrograded in the recent years, and the belief that fusimotor activity played no role on the progress of spasticity advanced [21].

### *Alteration of Cellular Levels*

Alterations of cellular levels develop secondary to the lesion. These secondary alterations may also be named as morphological plasticity. Plasticity develops from the healthy parts of partially denervated neurons in two forms: collateral sprouting and denervation super sensitivity [22]. Despite the lack of absolute proof, malplasticity is believed to contribute to the progress of spasticity in human beings and to have major effects particularly on the increased motor-neuron activation of alfa and gamma **motoneurons' denervation** super sensitivity.

### *Others*

Unmasking of silent spinal interneurons, presynaptic alterations [23], nonsynaptic changes in spinal neurons (serotinin, noreepinephrine), post-synaptic hypersensitivity (long-term potential) are the other inconclusive factors thought to have a role in the spinal mechanism of spasticity.

The neural component of spasticity eventuating through spinal mechanism is complicated and has inconclusive characteristics [24]. These neural and non-neural components are listed in Table 2.

Spasticity does not eventuate forth with spinal lesion. Determined by lesion intensity, lesion localization and individual differences, symptoms of spasticity occur gradually following the lesion. This period is often named as the "spinal shock phase." Why is there a silent period? The answer to this question is not clear enough. Spinal shock phase is thought to occur by reasons of alterations in the electrical activity of motor neurons—particularly gamma motorneurons— (hyperpolarization), denervation super sensitivity, etc. This model (presumption) is mostly effectual for acute traumatic cord injuries. The silent period does not occur in chronic diseases like MS.

Over the course of time, as the symptoms become chronic, neural component symptoms of spasticity are accompanied by non-neural component symptoms of spasticity. The non-neural component develops as a result of the increase in the intrinsic mechanical stiffness of the muscle. Studies support that sarcomere length and cellular elastic modulus of the spastic muscle differs from that of a healthy person [25, 26]. Furthermore, cohesive with immobilization, motor unit types undergo an alteration: type I fibers mutate to type II. This change is believed to be the result of unrelaxed spastic muscle (due to over activity), and—although reciprocal—more severe paresis in the antagonist muscle [24]. These alterations in the intrinsic structure of the spastic muscle screen the "velocity dependent involuntary resistance to passive movement" feature of spasticity, and the muscles become equally responsive to both fast and slow movements. Unless the alterations in the biomechanical structure of the muscle are contained, ROM becomes restricted followed by contractures over the course of time.

**Table 2. Pathophysiological mechanism of spasticity**

| Probable Mechanisms |
| --- |
| **Supraspinal changes** |
| Sprouting from undamaged descending pathways |
| **Spinal changes** |
| Increased alfa-MN excitability |
| Decreased presynaptic inhibition on Ia afferents |
| Decreased homosynaptic depression |
| Decreased Ib inhibition |
| Increased group II facilitory effects |
| Increased renshaw inhibition during contraction |
| Decreased Ia reciprocal inhibition during contraction |
| **Soft tissue changes** |
| Intrinsic muscle stiffness |

## 3.5. SUPRASPINAL MECHANISM OF SPASTICITY

Cerebral efficacy in MS usually occurs due to partial atrophies and axonal loss in several areas and in anatomically localized demyelinization plaques like corpus callosum, optic tractus, periventricular white matter, cerebellum and brain stem. Supraspinal mechanism of spasticity has both similar and dissimilar characteristics with hemiplegic spasticity, which occurs as an outcome of CVA.

Spasticity is conventionally defined as an upper motor neuron symptom developed as an outcome of pyramidal tractus lesion. Nonetheless, it is known that pyramidal tractus lesions, unaccompanied by other lesions, usually result in weakness effecting the distal; that they do not lead to hypertonus/hyperreflexia [27]. Therefore, it can be claimed that some parts of the cerebrum have an excitatory and some parts have an inhibitory effect on the muscle tonicity. Under normal conditions, there is a delicate balance between the excitatory/inhibitory effect.

Pyramidal tractus starts from the fourth cortical area—which is also known as the primary motor cortex. This area has a particular exciting effect on the distal muscle tonicity and activity. According to experimental studies on animals and clinical characteristics of human beings (pyramidal lesion is rarely seen separately—it usually develops during surgical operations), lesion in this area alone eliminate the excitatory effect and result in flask paralysis and hyporeflexia.

Premotor areas are localized in the areas six and eight of the cerebral cortex. These areas, particularly the supplementary motor area generating the parapyramidal system, are considered responsible for the regulation of muscle tonicity. This regulation is actualized in the form of controlling the increasing effect of primary cortex on muscle tonicity. In the case of a lesion affecting both pyramidal tractus and parapyramidal fibers starting from the premotor areas, spastic paralysis and hyperflexia occur [27].

Reticular formation located in the brain and pedunculus also has an essential effect on the regulation of muscle tonicity. Particularly, the dorsal bulbar reticular area has an inhibitory effect on muscle tonicity. Anterior and paramedian cerebellar cortex and fastigial nucleus also participate in the inhibition of bulbar reticular area. The bulbar reticular area needs to receive impulses from premotor cortical areas in order to accomplish its inhibitory task. Therefore, spasticity is an expected result when premotor areas are affected by the lesion, even if the bulbar reticular area is not affected [28, 29].

On the other hand, pons and pontine reticular system, which vestibular system originates from, have a facilitating effect on muscle tonicity. It generates this facilitating effect alone, without any stimulation from supraspinal centers. Pons and vestibulospinal activity have an important role in the progress of decerebration rigidity. Basal diencephelon, central grey and tegmentum of the midbrain and lateral bulbar reticular formation are the other areas with facilitating effects on muscle tonicity [27].

Spasticity generated with stroke and other similar pathologies in cortical and capsular patterns affect the antigravity muscles of the body, resulting in hypertonia in the flexor muscles of upper extremities and extansor muscles of lower extremities. This is an outcome of rub-rospinal tract (starting from the red nucleus in midbrain), facilitating the motor neurons of upper extremity flexor muscles and inhibiting the motoneurons of the extansor muscles. Ventromedial reticulaspinal tract has a similar effect. Vestibulospinal tract—on the other hand—sends facilitating impulses to the extansory motoneurons of lower body and lower extremity muscles and has inhibitory effects on flexor muscles [13].

Though a similar course may be seen in MS, hypertonia may occur in a more complicated way in unexpected muscle groups. This results from the localization of demyelization plaques.

## 3.6. OTHER CHARACTERISTICS OF SPASTICITY

### 3.6.1. Clasp Knife Phenomenon

When the extremity muscle is moved passively in the direction of the antagonist of spastic pattern, spastic muscle responds with a sudden resistance. If the extremity is held stabilized for a while at the spot of resistance, a sudden relaxation is observed in spastic muscle. This clinical feature of spasticity is called "clasp knife phenomenon." Time required for the relaxation of the muscle depends on the intensity of spasticity. The more intense the spasticity is, the slower clasp knife phenomenon may occur. In chronic cases with severe stiffness in the intrinsic structure of the muscle, spasticity may not occur at all.

When the muscle is held stretched, excitability of tonic stretch reflex decreases and a tension is loaded on the muscle, stimulates golgi tendon organs, and initiates autogenetic inhibition. This process is believed to be the cause of the clasp knife phenomenon [29].

### 3.6.2. Flexor Spasms

Flexor spasms may be observed in most of the spastic patients, causing more pain and discomfort than spasticity itself. Spasticity—studied pathophysiologically— develops independently from deep tendon reflexes and clonus. Therefore, flexor spasms are believed not to be dependent on abnormal proprioceptive reflexes as well. They are presumed to be the outcome of normal flexor withdrawal reflexes that have become disinhibited. Threshold of flexor withdrawal reflex decreases as a result of upper motor lesion. Afferent impulses sent from periphery skin, muscles, subcutaneous tissues and joints stimulate polysynaptic reflexes and cause spasms in flexor muscles. Elimination of the inhibitory effect of dorsal reticulospinal tract is believed to be influential in this process in particular [29]. According to clinical experiences, flexor spasms actualized through spinal mechanism are more common than that of supraspinal spasticity.

### 3.6.3. Associated Reactions

Associated reactions are involuntary inertias observed in wrist and finger flexors of patients while they are walking or performing a complicated activity. Associated reactions are remote forms of synkinesis and may be due to a failure to inhibit spread motor activity [28,30]. They are mostly observed in supraspinal lesions and increase in direct proportion with the intensity of spasticity.

Independent from anatomical levels, upper motor lesions cause functional disorders in patients by creating a vicious circle of positive and negative symptoms.

Composed of complex findings altogether, a number of characteristics of spasticity still remain unclear. As studies in this area continue, the unclear aspects will be clarified and, perhaps, new and more satisfactory data will lead us and clinicians to different directions in managing spasticity. The most important thing that has to be done on the basis of our current knowledge is to assess an MS patient on several grounds and from many aspects. This is important mostly in the selection and application of appropriate physical therapy techniques used in the management of spasticity.

## 3.7. CONCLUSION

Anatomical structures such as cerebrum, cerebellum, and spinal cord are affected and UMN symptoms—along with other symptoms—are generated in MS, among which, spasticity develops both with spinal and supraspinal mechanisms.

Definition of spasticity differs according to disciplinary viewpoints within the rehabilitation team. Neurologists and physicians regard spasticity as a clinical finding, as increased muscle tone marked by "exaggerated tendon jerks" and "excessive tonic reflexes," whereas physiotherapists refer to spasticity through its functional aspects.

Normal motor movement is actualized by spinal reflexes functioning under the modulation and control of upper centers. Formation of spinal reflexes requires impulses generated by proprioceptors such as muscle fiber, golgi tendon organ, etc. Golgi tendon organ is active during the maximal contraction of the muscle, whereas muscle fiber is active when the muscle is in its most stretched position. These physiological features are important for the physical therapist while applying muscle inhibition and facilitation techniques.

The physiotherapist should have a profound theoretical knowledge of spasticity and be able to collate his theoretical knowledge with the practical one relying on his personal clinical experiences. Thereby, he would foresee probable symptoms and findings of a spastic patient, enabling him to save both his and his patient's time and energy during the clinical assessments.

## 3.8. REFERENCES

[1]	Lance, J.W. (1980). Symposium synopsis. In Feldman R.G. & Young R.R.& Koella W.P (eds.), *Spasticity disorders of motor control* (edition 1, pp. 485-494 ), Chicago: Year Book Medical Publisher.
[2]	Sköld, C. & Levi R. & Seiger A. (1999). Spasticity after traumatic spinal cord injury: nature, severity, and location. *Arch Phys Med Rehabil,* 80, 1548-1557
[3]	Dietz, V.(2000). Spastic movement disorder. *Spinal Cor, 38,* 389-393.
[4]	Bohannon, RW. (1993). Tilt table standing for reducing spasticity after spinal cord injury. *Arch Phys Med Rehabil,* 74, 1121-1122.
[5]	Kita, M. & Goodkin, DE. (2000). Drugs used to treat spasticity. *Drugs, 59,* 487-495.
[6]	Young, R.R. (1994).Spasticity: a review. *Neurology,* 44 (suppl 9):S12-S20.
[7]	Bernstein, N. (1967). The coordination and regulation of movement. Oxford, Pergamon Press.
[8]	Shakespeare, D.T. & Craig, J. & Lloyd, M. (2001). Spasticity and Movement. *The intern MS journ,* 7, no: 93-99.
[9]	Satkunam, L.E. (2003). Rehabilitation medicine: 3. Management of adult spasticity. *CMAJ,* 169(11), 1173-1179.
[10]	Knutsson, E. & Richards, C. (1979). Different types of disturbed motor control in gait of hemiparetic patients. *Brain,* 102:405-430.
[11]	Bear, M.F. & Connors, B.W.& Paradiso M.A. (2001). *Neuroscience: Exploring the Brain.* (2.edition). Baltimore, Maryland: Lippincott Williams &Wilkins: A Wolter Kluwer Company.
[12]	Stevenson, V.L. & Louise, J. (2006). *Spasticity management: a practical multidisciplinary guide* (edition 1). Oxon: İnforma Healthcare
[13]	Biering Sorensen, F. & Nielsen, J.B. & Klinge, K. (2006). Spasticity assessment: a review. *Spinal Cord,* 44(12), 708-722.
[14]	Crone, C. & Nielsen J. (1994). Central control of disynaptic reciprocal inhibition in humans. *Acta Physiol Scand,* 152,351-363.

[15]  Gelber, A. & Douglas, R.F. (2002). *Clinical evaluation and management of spasticity* (1 edition). Totowa, New Jersey: Humana Press.

[16]  Katz, R. & Pierrot, D.E. (1982). Recurrent inhibition of alpha-motoneurons in patients with upper motor neuron lesions. *Brain,* 57, 103-124.

[17]  Katz, R. & Pierrot, D.E. (1999). Recurrent inhibition in humans. *Prog Neurobiol,* 57, 325-355.

[18]  Mazzocchio, R. & Rossi, A. (1989). Recurrent inhibition in human spinal spasticity. *Ital Neurol Sci,* 10, 337-347.

[19]  Raynor, E.M. & Shefner, JM. (1994). Recurrent inhibition is decreased in patients with amyotrophic lateral sclerosis. *Neurology,* 44, 2148-2150.

[20]  Hultborn, H. & Brownstone, R.B.& Toth T.I.& Gossard J.P. (2004). Key mechanisms for setting the input-output gain across the motoneuron pool. *Prog Brain Res* 143, 77-95.

[21]  Nielsen, J.B. & Crone, C.& Hultborn, H. (2007). The spinal pathophysiology of spasticity—from a basic science point of view. *Acta Physiol (Oxf),* 189(2), 171-80.

[22]  Bareyre, F.M. & Kerschensteiner, M. & Raineteau, O.& Mettenleiter, T.C. & Weinmann, O.& Schwab, M.E. (2004). The injured spinal cord spontaneously forms a new intraspinal circuit in adult rats. *Nat Neurosci,* 7, 269-277.

[23]  Delwaide, P.J. & Olivier, E (1988). Short-latency autogenic inhibition (IB inhibition) in human spasticity. *J Neurol Neurosurg Psychiatry,* 51, 1546-1550.

[24]  Gracies, J.M. (2005). Pathophysiology of spastic paresis. II: Emergence of muscle over activity. *Muscle Nerve,* 31(5),552-571.

[25]  Lieber, R.L. & Steinman, S. & Barash, I.A. & Chambers H. (2004). Structural and functional changes in spastic skeletal muscle. *Muscle Nerve,* 29(5), 615-627.

[26]  Foran, J.R. & Steinman, S. & Barash, I. Chambers, H.G. & Lieber, R.L. (2005). Structural and mechanical alterations in spastic skeletal muscle. *Dev Med Child Neurol,* 47(10), 713-717.

[27]  Brown, P. (1994). Pathophysiology of spasticity. *J Neurol Neurosurg Psychiatry,* 57, 773-777.

[28]  Guyton, A.C. & Hall J.E. (1995). *Text book of medical physiology* (edition 9). Michigan: W. Saunders.

[29]  Sheean, G. (2002).The pathophysiology of spasticity. *Eur J Neurol,* 9 (Suppl 1):3-9, 53-61.

[30] Macfarlane A, Turner-Stokes L, De Souza L. (2002). The associated
     reaction rating scale: a clinical tool to measure associated reactions in the
     hemiplegic upper limb. *Clin Rehabil.* 16(7):726-35.

*Chapter 4*

# MS AND SPASTICITY

## Kadriye Armutlu[*]

Hacettepe University, Faculty of Health Sciences, Department of Physical
Therapy and Rehabilitation, Neurological Rehabilitation Unit
06100/Ankara/TURKEY

## 4.1. ABSTRACT

Spasticity is a common problem among patients with MS, and the rate is
presumed to be between 40 to 75%. According to some of resources, this rate
is as high as 84%. Spasticity causes fatigue, painful spasms, contractures,
gait abnormalities, poor mobility and secondary strength loss in antagonist
muscles. Spasticity and its intensity may alter due to infections, urine
retentions, bladder or kidney stones, constipations, skin ulcerations, nail
immersions, usage of incompetible orthesis, inappropriate positions in bed or
wheelchair and tight clothing.

MS treatment becomes more complex and difficult when the disease is
present with the spasticity. The aim of physical therapy in MS must be
reducing aggravation of other symptoms such as weakness, fatigue, painful
spasms and inducing mobility level of patients by managing spasticity and
modulating hypertonus.

Key words: Multiple sclerosis, spasticity, walking, mobility, functions.

---

* Email: karmutlu@hacettepe.edu.tr

## 4.2. INTRODUCTION

Spasticity is a common problem among patients with MS. The symptom increases the intensity of defects MS patients experience, exposing itself by: causing secondary strength loss in antagonist muscles, fatigue—due to excessive energy consumption—painful spasms, contractures extending to restricted range of joint motion (ROM), gait abnormalities and poor mobility.

Spasticity is a disorder revealed when the spinal cord and/or brain is affected. The rate of spasticity in SCI is 65 to 78% and 35% in stroke incidents [1]; whereas the rate of spasticity in MS patients is higher since MS affects both the brain and the spinal cord [2, 3]. Spasticity rate in MS is presumed to be between 40 to 75% [4, 5, 6]. According to some other resources, this rate is as high as 84% [7]. This rate proves spasticity to be the second most common MS symptom following fatigue [5]. However, the number of studies concerning the outcomes and prevalence of spasticity and disabilities caused by spasticity is quite few [8].

## 4.3. CHARACTERISTICS AND ADVERSE EFFECTS OF SPASTISITY IN MS PATIENTS

When defined as a resistance to passive movement, the most common symptom of spasticity defined by patients is muscle stiffness together with painful spasms. According to this research, 64% of 74% patients with spasticity have muscle stiffness complaints, 51% have muscle spasm complaints and 74% have both muscle stiffness and muscle spasm complaints. Eighty percent of the patients who have taken part in this research have spasticity [5].

In the light of clinical experiences, MS spasticity is observed to start in the lower extremity distal—particularly in the triceps surae muscles—and generally exceeding to the quadriceps femoris [9]. In the following phases, hip adductors and gluteus maximus may be affected by spasticity. In progressive MS cases with severe demiyelinization and axonal loss in spinal cord, hamstring muscle group may rarely be affected as well. According to EDSS, influenced by the duration of the disease and the intensity of the defect, upper extremity starts at the level of 6.5 to 7 and generally includes the flexor muscles of the finger and wrist.

Clinical experiences show that the intensity of painful muscle spasms increases by the severity of spasticity are in direct proportion with intensity of spasticity. Patients with moderate spasticity convey that they feel their legs so stiff that they are unable to move them when they wake up; however, the stiffness subsides with activation but recurs with continued movements (i.e., walking); on the contrary, in mild spasticity, stiffness generally exposes itself not during rest but with activation, and its severity rises relatively particularly during walking.

The most extensive research about spasticity is made by Rizzo et al., covering the frequency and the distribution of spasticity according to subtypes and symptom duration, its characteristics and its impacts on patient's quality of life. According to the findings of this particular research applied to 21,000 patients registered to The North American Research Committee on MS, 16% of patients have no spasticity, 31% have minimal, 19% have mild (occasional), 17% have moderate (frequently affects activities), 13% have severe (need to modify daily activities) and 4% have drastically severe (prevents daily activities) spasticities [10]. As is known, when the male patients of declining age are considered, the activation of the MS syndrome is higher and the defects are more severe. One of the most fundamental outcomes of this research is about gender differences. Male patients mostly took place in the "drastically severe spasticity" group. Another outcome of the experiment is that patients with severe spasticity had longer disease duration while their MS symptoms regressed and had attacks during the research period. As a conclusion, it is clear that no matter which type of MS, there is a direct linear relationship between the disease activation and spasticity [10].

Disease occurrence rate and its intensity are determined by the subtype and activation of the disease. More than the half of the stabilized RRMS-type patients have no complaints of spasticity. On the other hand, though in the relapsing type, among patients with high disease activation, the frequency and severity of spasticity increases meaningfully. Although the number of patients with PPMS type is minimum, the rate of spasticity is very high [10].

Despite the limited number of verified data present, it is believed that there is an inferential correlation between the presence and severity of spasticity and the cognitive level of the patient. This relationship may be explained by spasticity's effect on increasing fatigue, which, in return, leads to cognitive weariness resulting in deterioration of the cognitive processes level of the patient.

Independent of the type of MS, its severity and activation, medication use is effective on the progress and intensity of spasticity as well. Despite the contradicting opinions, long-term usage of beta interferon increases the intensity of spasticity [11].

Spasticity is an important factor in aggravating the severity of defects and disabilities in MS patients. Spasticity's complicating effects, especially on walking, occur due to over consumption of energy, fatigue and an increase in bladder problems. According to the findings of Rizzo et al., the patients' points ascend in The Patient Determined Disease Step in parallel with increasing problems in walking; while their points in scales like SF-36 evaluating the quality of life decrease concurrently with spasticity [10].

Spasticity is severe in the active progressive types of MS. The ambulation of the patient is made possible with at least one crutch, and when the spasticity severity level is two or more. In cases of drastic severe types and total spasticity, the patient has to use a wheelchair in order to ambulate [10]. Even the act of transferring the patient to the wheelchair is a problematic process in severe spasticity cases [12].

In addition to spasticity's negative effects on mobilization and walking activity of the patient, it causes frequent falls resulting in orthopedical problems.

According to a study conducted by Peterson et al. on 354 MS patients, 50% of subjects had injurious fall histories [13].

Frequent falls in MS patients bring about the risk of fractures. Immunosuppressive treatment, involving steroid application, may cause bone osteoporosis [14, 15].

Although osteoblastics are applied to these patients in order to maintain normal bone density level and support bones, osteoporosis cannot be obstructed, resulting in the risk of fractures as an ongoing and common problem among MS patients.

Nilsagard et al., who thought that falls and factors aggrevating the risk of fractures should be surveyed, conducted a study on 76 MS patients who have EDSS scores between 3.5 to 6. Statistical differences in symptoms observed between patients with fall complaints and patients who do not have fall complaints can be listed as: spasticity, proprioception and ataxia [16].

According to clinical experiences and statements of patients, the major factor in deteriorating patient's quality of life is poor mobility resulting from the features of spasticity [17] and its interaction with other MS symptoms, leading to the formation of a vicious circle (schematized in figure 1).

Pyramidal symptoms and existence of spasticity (being a major symptom) in lower extremities aggravate bladder problems [18,19]. Spasticity has a negative outcome on sexual activities for both gender groups (especially on female patients), affecting the hip adductors. Furthermore, patients with severe adductor spasticity complain about having problems in hygiene and skin care, demanding a third person's assistance in such matters.

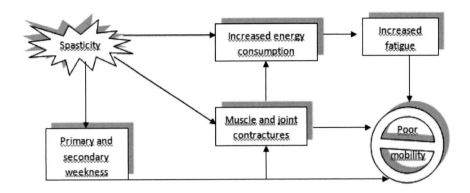

Figure 1. Schematization of factors causing poor mobility.

Occasionally, unexpected complications of spasticity may arise. Patedjl et al. reported such a case in 2008. The subject was a 63-year-old PPMS patient with severe spasticity particularly in lower extremity suffering from tetraparesis. Due to secondary low extremity weakness, the patient was able to take a few steps with a walker and by reason of extensory spasticity in legs, she was only able to stabilize in standing position. According to Ashworth Scale (AS), she had three to four degrees of spasticity in her hip adductors, resulting in pain and distress during nighttime. When application of Baclofen did not help in managing spasticity, she was injected with botilinum toxin type A, which also did not work, whereupon the decision was made to apply triamcinolone acetonide (Volon A®) intrathecally; however, when the patient was put in lumbar puncture position for the application, she had a sudden and severe pain and spasm in her femoris lasting for long hours. When the area was scanned with sonography, a longitudinal rupture and hematoma in her left adductor muscle **was detected. The patient's** spasticity was managed by use of intrathecal medication and physical therapy applications. Although during follow-up examinations the sonographic images showed some residual hematoma, the patient was pain free to some account [20].

While the spasticity can lead to series of unexpected side effects as the above-mentioned literature indicates, it can rarely come to existence as complication of some treatment techniques as well. In addition to that, it can be present in unexpected muscle groups that represent an unexpected clinical picture. Hereby, we present two case stories briefly that we followed in our clinic:

**CASE 1**

Mr. X is a 48-year–old, single male engineer, who was diagnosed with MS 12 years ago at his first visit to his neurologist with the balance problems. The disease began and progressed as RRMS form of MS during the first four to five years. Later on, it turned to SPMS form of MS, which lead to the severe cerebellar problems. Although patient did not have any spasticity problems, he was not able to use his right hand due to progressing tremors. Meanwhile, he used Rivotril (klonazepam) as a medication along with the physical therapy. However, his cerebellar symptoms increased severely by time. For that reason, the decision of a tremor surgery was taken. After the application of sterotactic talamotomy surgery, his tremors decreased obviously. However, hemiparesis developed in the right half of the entire body. After the surgery, the spasticity that is changing between 1 + and 2 during rest and increasing with the physical effort developed, according to MAS measurement in quadriceps femoris, tibialis posterior and gluteal muscles in the right lower extremity. On the other hand, the balance was not affected at all. In addition to the mentioned situations, thalamic hand posture came to existence in his right hand. At the moment, patient is continuing to use Rivotril and Sirdalud as medication. In addition to that, he has botilinum toxin applications to his gastro-soleus, tibialis posterior and long finger flexors with the periods of 4-5 months, near by the regular physical therapy (figure 2).

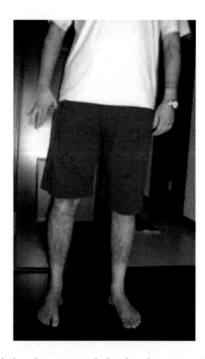

Figure 2. Case 1 (thalamic hand posture and plantigrade response).

---

**CASE 2**

Mrs. Y is a 58-year-old, retired female who was diagnosed with MS 18 years ago. The disease began as RRMS form of MS, which became SPMS form later on. The disease shows itself with the spasticity in distal lower extremities and the balance problems since the first years of its occurrence. Patient mentions that her lumbar extensors feels harder, she cannot stand straight due to this stiff and painful feeling and has difficulties during gait for the last three to four years. L4-5 disc herniation was seen in his MRI; however, it did not require a surgery due to its level. Therefore, it was assumed that the stiffness and the pain in his lower back were triggered by the disc herniation. Although oral muscle relaxants were used, low back area was irresponsive to the medication. Thus botulinum toxin application was considered, however patient did not accept the application. For that reason a physical therapy programme that is arranged for the general symptom management began to be used, focusing mainly on the low back area. At the moment, patient is quite responsive to prolonged ice application and to soft tissue and joint mobilization techniques and his physical therapy goes on regularly.

---

## 4.4. FACTORS AGGRAVATING THE SEVERITY OF SPASTICITY

Spasticity and its intensity may alter temporarily during the day due to a number of reasons such as: bladder infections/other infections, urine retentions, bladder/kidney stones, constipations, skin ulcerations, nail immersions, usage of incompetible orthesis, improper wheelchair/bed positions and tight clothing [21]. Increase in body and/or room temperature may temporarily aggravate spasticity in MS Patients.

## 4.5. CONCLUSION

Spasticity is quite a common symptom of MS, with the rate of 84%. With the addition of spasticity to numerous other symptoms caused by MS, the disease becomes more complex. Spasticity leads to problems in most of the patient's activities, particularly in mobility. Hip adductor spasticity, in particular, has a negative effect on hygiene and skin-care.

In early phases of MS, physiotherapist usually deals with minimal and mild spasticity developed in distal lower extremity. Most affected muscle groups are m. gastro-soleus, m. quadriceps femoris, m. guluteus maximus. In situations where spasticity is generated in spinal cord, hip adductors and hamstring muscle groups are affected. Spasticity in upper extremities is observed in the advanced phases of the disease (EDSS≥6.5 to 7).

Depending on MS subtypes, spasticity is more severe and frequent in patients with progressive type of MS, whereas its frequency and severity is less in patients with RRMS. However, spasticity is aggravated during relapses.

Spasticity aggravates the severity of symptoms like fatigue, weakness, bladder and sexual problems.

Treatment determined by the physiotherapist should target the management of spasticity and indirect modulation of hypertonus through the application of methods designed to moderate spasticity's **aggravating effect on the other** symptoms. Such an approach is fundamental for patients whose spasticity, along with mobility problems, has negative effects on their personal and social lives.

## 4.6. REFERENCES

[1]    Haselkorn, J.K. & Loomis, S. (2005). Multiple sclerosis and spasticity. *Phys Med Rehabil Clin N Am*, 16(2), 467-481.

[2]    Sommerfeld, D.K. & Eek, E.U. & Svensson A.K. & Holmqvist L.W. & Von Arbin M.H. (2004). Spasticity after stroke: its occurrence and association with motor impairments and activity limitations. *Stroke,* 35(1), 134-139.

[3]    Maynard, F.M & Karunas, R.S. & Waring W.P. (1990). 3rd. Epidemiology of spasticity following traumatic spinal cord injury. *Arch Phys Med Rehabil,* 71(8), 566-569.

[4]    Brar, S.P. & Smith, M.B. & Nelson L.M. & Franklin G.M. & Cobble N.D. (1991). Evaluation of treatment protocols on minimal to moderate spasticity in multiple sclerosis. *Arch Phys Med Rehabil,* 72(3), 186-189.

[5]    Paisley, S. & Beard, S. & Hunn A & Wight J. (2002) Clinical effectiveness of oral treatments for spasticity in multiple sclerosis: a systematic review. *Mult Scler,* 8(4), 319-329.

[6]    Smith, C.R. & LaRocca, N.G. & Giesser, B.S. & Scheinberg, L.C. (1991). High-dose oral baclofen: experience in patients with multiple sclerosis. *Neurology,* 41: 1829-1831.

[7]    Collin, C. & Davies, P. & Mutiboko I.K. & Ratcliffe S. (2007). Sativex Spasticity in MS Study Group. Randomized controlled trial of cannabis-

based medicine in spasticity caused by multiple sclerosis. *Eur J Neurol*, 14(3), 290-296.

[8]   Crayton, H.J. & Rossman, H.S. (2006). Managing the symptoms of multiple sclerosis: a multimodal approach. *Clin Ther*. 28(4):445-60.

[9]   Kesselring, J. (1999). Long-term management and rehabilitation in multiple sclerosis. In Siva A.& Kesselring J. & Thompson A.J (eds.), *Frontiers in Multiple Sclerosis Volume 2* (edition 2, pp. 234-252), London: Martin Dunitz.

[10]  Rizzo, M.A. & Hadjimichael, O.C. & Preiningerova , J. & Vollmer T.L. (2004). Prevalence and treatment of spasticity reported by multiple sclerosis patients. *Mult Scler*, 10(5), 589-595.

[11]  Walther, E.U. & Hohlfeld, R. (1999). Multiple sclerosis: side effects of interferon beta therapy and their management. Neur*ology*,10;53(8),1622-1627.

[12]  Boissy, A.R. & Cohen, J.A. (2007). Multiple sclerosis symptom management. *Expert Rev Neurother*, 7(9),1213-1222.

[13]  Peterson, E.W. & Cho, C.C. & von Koch, L. & Finlayson, M.L. (2008). Injurious falls among middle-aged and older adults with multiple sclerosis. *Arch Phys Med Rehabil*. 89(6):1031-7.

[14]  Faulkner, M.A. & Ryan-Haddad, A.M. & Lenz, T.L. & Degner, K.(2005). Osteoporosis in long-term care residents with multiple sclerosis. *Consult Pharm*, 20(2):128-36.).

[15]  Zorzon, M.& Zivadinov, R. & Locatelli, L. & Giuntini, D. & Toncic, M. & Bosco, A.& Nasuelli, D. & Bratina, A. & Tommasi, M.A. & Rudick, R.A. & Cazzato, G. (2005). Long-term effects of intravenous high-dose methylprednisolone pulses on bone mineral density in patients with multiple sclerosis. *Eur J Neurol*, 12 (7):550-6.

[16]  Nilsagård, Y. & Lundholm, C. & Denison, E. & Gunnarsson, L.G. (2008). Predicting accidental falls in people with multiple sclerosis—a longitudinal study. *J Neurol*, 255 Suppl 6:115-8.

[17]  Freeman JA. (2001). Improving mobility and functional independence in persons with multiple sclerosis. *J Neurol*. 248(4):255-9. Review.

[18]  Betts, C.D. & D'Mellow, M.T. & Fowler, C.J. (1993). Urinary symptoms and the neurological features of bladder dysfunction in multiple sclerosis. *J Neurol Neurosurg Psychiatry*, 56(3), 245-250.

[19]  Valleroy, M.L & Kraft, G.H. (1984). Sexual dysfunction in multiple sclerosis. *Arch Phys Med Rehabil*, 65(3), 125-128.

[20] Patejdl, R. & Winkelmann, A. & Benecke, R. & Zettl, U.K. (2008). Muscle rupture caused by exacerbated spasticity in a patient with multiple sclerosis. *J Neurol,* 255 Suppl 6:115-8.)

[21] Satkunam, L.E. (2003). Rehabilitation medicine: 3. Management of adult spasticity. *CMAJ,* 169(11), 1173-1179.

In: Spasticity and Its Management ...
Editor: Kadriye Armutlu

ISBN: 978-1-60876-185-5
© 2010 Nova Science Publishers, Inc.

*Chapter 5*

# POSTURE AND BODY MECHANICS

## *Kadriye Armutlu**

Hacettepe University, Faculty of Health Sciences, Department of Physical
Therapy and Rehabilitation, Neurological Rehabilitation Unit
06100/Ankara/TURKEY

## 5.1. ABSTRACT

The human body has quite a flexible and multisegmental structure. Movements of body segments are quite different from one another. Gravitational forces act on all particles in a mass, especially the centre of gravity defined as the point at which the sum of all moments is equal to zero and is the point at which the body is balanced. Spasticity causes misalignment of joint and muscles resulting in alterations in body mechanics. Spasticity also may cause bad posture and weakness muscles. To reduce this bad posture may help spasticity management, the Alexander Technique, the Feldenkrais method and Pilates can be used to correct posture.

Key words: posture, body mechanics, postural management, alternative therapy techniques.

---

* Email: karmutlu@hacettepe.edu.tr

## 5.2. INTRODUCTION

Spasticity causes misalignment of joint and muscles resulting in alterations in body mechanics. The human body has quite a flexible and multisegmental structure. Flexibility enables maintenance of balance while in unexpected positions; various postural adaptations required for different activities may be actualized within the flexibility limits.

According to Whitman, erect posture is one's constant resistance to gravity. In more detailed terms, posture is to [1]:

- Conform to the supporting surface in terms of symmetry and equality of weight-bearing and contact surfaces;
- Select and adopt the alignment of body segments appropriate to the efficient performance of a chosen activity;
- Balance and stabilize the selected body attitude relative to the supporting surface;
- Adjust to changes within the body or support while maintaining balance and stability throughout the disturbance;
- Free from weight-bearing those parts of the body required for movement;
- Form reliable support for muscular movements.

## 5.3. BODY SEGMENTS AND THEIR MOVEMENTS

Head, thorax, pelvis, thighs, lower legs and feet are the main body segments. Head, pelvis and long bones are relatively rigid components. Connective tissues are spine, hip, knee, ankle and shoulder joints. The head is heavier in proportion to other segments and is balanced on the highly flexible cervical spine. The upper limb segment is additional weight carried by the trunk. The loading on the spine will increase or decrease according to the position of the arms at a given time.

Movements of body segments are quite different from one another. When surveyed as a whole, it is observed that the spinal column allows forward-flexion movement whereas extensions, lateral flexions and rotations are limited. These movements are actualized through joint movements between vertebrae. The movements between vertebrae are complex, combining flexion, rotation and gliding.

Hips and shoulders, which are pivot joints, create multi-planar movements controlled by muscles. The shoulder joint ligaments rely on the soft tissues for stability and, in cases of diminished or absent muscle control, these connecting tissues are particularly vulnerable to damage in handling. When compared to shoulder joint, movements of knee and ankle joints are quite limited. The two joints must be stabile since they carry the whole body weight [2].

In a sitting position, the hip and pelvis form the basis. The superficial structure above the pelvis is balanced on the rockers formed by the ischial and pubic rami, the whole rotating about the highly mobile pivot joint of the hip. Sagittal movement of the pelvis is limited only by contact of trunk with thigh in flexion and the tension of soft tissues in extension. In cases of poor muscle control, the pelvis rocks forth and back due to the effective forces. In pathologies like spasticity, which creates imbalance, fixation in a specific position is observed, which usually is the retraction of pelvis.

## 5.3.1. Gravitational Factors and Their Effects on Posture

Gravitational forces act on all particles in a mass, but have the net effect of acting at only one point, which is the centre of that mass or the centre of gravity. The centre of gravity may be defined as the point at which the sum of all moments is equal to zero and is the point at which the body is balanced.

Gravitational force actualizes with center of gravity and localization of line of gravity within the body. Under normal circumstances, the center of gravity is located in the anterior part of the second sacral vertebra. The gravity line passes through specific points of the body when a stabilized standing position is maintained. When persons with normal posture are analyzed laterally, the line should pass through the center of earlobe, shoulder joint and trochanter major, frontal part of thoracal vertebras, back of patella and 2 to 2.5 cm forward of lateral malleolus [3,4,5,6,7] (figure 1). Alterations in these values indicate balances with anterior or posterior glides. In a posterior analysis of posture, the gravity line should pass through the centre of spinal column and intergluteal cleavage and end in the centre of the support surface (figure 2). Alterations in these values mark balances with anterior or posterior glides as well.

Gravitational forces have activating and deactivating effects on muscles. For instance, m. quadriceps femoris is located before the gravity line in stabile standing position; therefore, the muscle has to be active in order to lock the knee joint. When the patient glides his body weight slightly forward, the gravity line is placed before the knee; the joint is mechanically locked without the tonic contraction of quadriceps femoris.

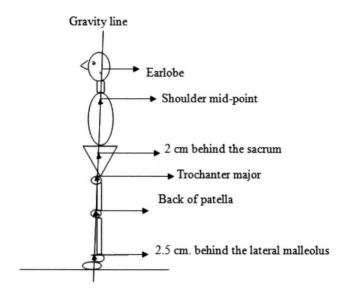

Figure 1. Lateral view of normal postural alignment in standing.

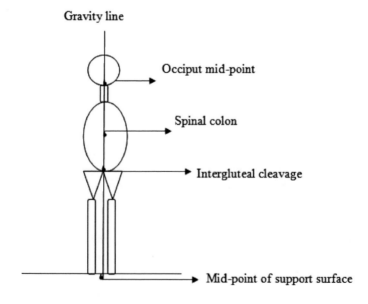

Figure 2. Posterior view normal postural alignment in standing.

Most patients who are subject to neurological diseases, MS in particular, spontaneously (unconsciously) glide their body weight towards anterior in order to generate a mechanical compensation of the weakened quadriceps femoris. Unused spastic quadriceps femoris gradually loses strength and shrinks. When the patient realizes that his knee is no longer capable of carrying his body weight, he avoids gliding his balance backwards and usually tries to lean forward, creating a vicious circle resulting in further impairment of the spastic muscle. During this process, m.gastrosoleus glides forward in constant contraction in order to maintain the balance and keep the body from falling. Spasticity is commonly observed in gastrosoleus. The muscle exercises maximum strength in static positions leading to shrinkage in its length and limitation in ankle ROM. If the foot is placed in inversion position with the shrinkage of m.tibialis posterior, the vicious circle of knee joint will aggravate.

This vicious circle begins to affect other joints as it moves forward from distal to proximal.

- Resulting from the gravity line that has glided forward, hip flexors are inactivated and, in patients with neurological deficits, this inactivation leads to further weakening of hip flexors.
- Pelvis gradually retracts as a result of weakened hip extensors with insufficient activation.
- In order to compensate for this situation, lumbar lordosis may aggravate.
- With the aggravation of lumbar lordosis, abdominal muscles weaken and lumbar extensors shorten.
- To compensate aggravated lumbar lordosis, throcal kyphosis may aggravate.
- Aggravated kyphotic posture causes weakness in paravertebral muscles that have been kept in a prolonged stretched position.
- In order to compensate throcal kyphos, cervical lordosis may aggravate, resulting in shrinkage of cervical vertebral muscles and gradual loss of strength in neck extensors.

## 5.3.2. The Effects of Bad Posture on Body Tissues and Nervous System

Not only joints and muscles but also connective and nervous tissues and lungs are negatively affected by the alterations in body segments. Due to bad posture, tissues of joint ligaments lose their connectivity features and gradually fail to act as supporters. Proprioceptors in ligaments that contribute to the creation of joint position sense eventually lose their sensitivity. Decrease in joint position sense has negative effects on patient's awareness of bad posture and his efforts to correct it.

The nervous system is a complementary structure and tension in a specific point causes pathologies within the whole system. For instance, most people are unaware of the important outcomes of kyphotic posture in a sitting position. While sitting in a kyphotic posture for long durations (sitting in class, watching tv, etc.), the head is in hyperextension position in order to adjust visual angle. Sympathetic truncus—a sympathetic component of autonomous nervous system, which is an important part of central nervous system—is located on both sides of vertebral column. It is located slightly lateral caudal in throcal area and lateral cranial in cervical area. Kyphotic posture stiffens the throcal part of the sympathetic truncus. Meanwhile, due to the hyperextension of the head, neck flexors and sympathetic truncus in cervical area are both subject to tension (figures 3 and 4). Tension of sympathetic truncus on both sides triggers sympathetic occurrences and the person begins to feel tense; muscle tone increases around the neck and shoulders; he may even have tachycardia. The extensive effects of this posture even on healthy people calls for an emphasis on the outcomes of bad posture on patients with spasticity and neurological deficits.

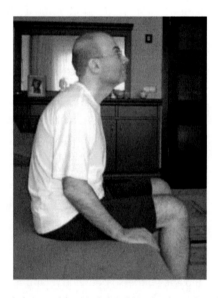

Figure 3: Bad posture in sitting position (minimal kyphosis and neck hyperextension).

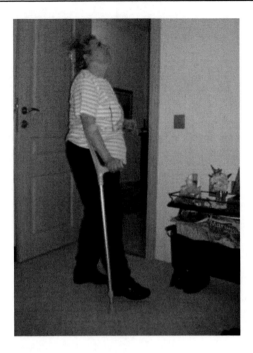

Figure 4: Bad posture in walking (neck hyperextension).

A common problem among patients with neurological deficits arises from the use of weak flexor muscles contrary to spastic extensory muscles of low extremities while walking. During each step, the patient spontaneously raises his shoulders and places his head into hyperextension in order to derive strength. This effort spent during each step may stimulate sympathetic nervous system and aggravate hypertonus.

Kyphotic and scoliotic posture has negative effects on lungs as well. Bad posture deteriorates the compliance and ventilation of lungs, which are under mechanical pressure locally. Due to poor ventilation—along with other factors, — lungs will be more receptive to infections. Such cases may shorten the lifespan of patients with chronic progressive diseases such as MS.

## 5.4. METHODS OF POSTURAL MANAGEMENT

The method of postural management (active exercises applied by the patient himself or manual applications of the physical therapist or orthoses) is determined by the severity of postural defects and impairment level of the patient. What should be kept in mind is that pelvis constitutes the key point in postural management, and the process should be initialized from this point on. The sequence listed below should be followed in postural management [2]:

- Primarily, pelvis asymmetries and pelvic posture defects in sitting position should be corrected. Patients with neurological deficits place their body weight on ischium instead of sacrum while sitting, resulting in the development of posterior pelvic tilt in sitting position, which aggravates throcal kyphos. The patient should be instructed to contract transversus abdominous in order to develop pelvis stabilization. Moreover, the physiotherapist should try to restore the original length of stretched and contracted structures.
- Subsequently, the ankle—a body segment of major importance—should be managed. Inversion and plantar flexion pattern should be averted with external support in the sitting position. Feet should contact the ground and be placed in a proper angle. In a standing position, inversion should be checked and reduced. To reduce the inversion, a lateral wedge insole may be applied. Unless this problem is averted, the ankle will be receptive to injuries and management of the knee will not be actualized.
- Hyperextension of the knee causes genu recurvatum, resulting in knee cartilage damage and pain. Uncontrolled hyperextension of the knee cannot be averted if the ankle stays in plantar flexion and inversion. In a sitting position, knees should be placed in parallel to each other with a 90° angle.
- Thighs should be placed parallel to each other in a slight abduction and neutral rotation. When decontrolled, thighs incur external rotation with the effect of gravity. External supports may be used in order to avoid such a case. In addition, crossing the legs several times a day averts extensory thrust and maintains tensor facialata in stretched position.
- The back of patient should be supported in a sitting position; there should be no lateral flexion and rotation in the trunk. If the patient has a tendency to sit on sacrum (lumbar lordosis is reversed in patients sitting on sacrum), a pillow should be placed at the waist to create pushing effect in lumbar lordosis direction. Arms should be supported; they should not swing at the sides.
- If there is increased cervical lordosis, the patient should be taught how to perform cervical stabilization exercises and be supported with a collar, if necessary.

## 5.5. ALTRENATIVE THERAPY TECHNIQUES TO RE-EDUCATE POSTURE

For patients who are able to participate in exercises actively (early and mid-phase MS), there are several training techniques developed for the improvement of postural control and awareness. Among these, the Alexander Technique, the Feldenkrais method and Pilates are highly common. Features of these techniques are summed up below.

### 5.5.1. The Alexander Technique

This technique was formulated almost 100 years ago by the Australian actor Frederick Matthias Alexander. He suffered from chronic vocal hoarseness when performing and was little helped by medical treatment or vocal training. Alexander decided to try to solve the problem himself by observing himself in specifically positioned mirrors. He noticed that he tended to pull his head back and down and was convinced that this was the cause of his problems. Alexander believed that the head, neck and body were interconnected and that whatever was done with one area of the body inevitably affected other areas. He forced himself to dissociate from what felt natural and right and to learn new habits by conscious effort.

Alexander developed his theory to include the concept that the spine is where "primary control" lies. In order to function properly, the spine must be lengthened not compressed, as shortening of the spine puts undue strain on all limbs and organs. The neck should always be free of tension, as tension will spread from there throughout the body. The head should be held forward and up and torso should be allowed to lengthen and widen out. With practice, the new ways of holding the body will lead to new sensory experience and unconscious bad habits will be replaced. Alexander also preached the need for proper breathing but never formulated a set of breathing exercises as such [8,9,10,11,12].

### 5.5.2. The Feldenkrais Method

Dr Moshe Feldenkrais developed a method of self-observation and learning following a serious leg injury. He studied his habitual way of moving and became aware of how limiting this was. Feldenkrais worked on methods to teach people how to learn about their bodies, developing two techniques, "awareness through movement" and "functional integration" [13,14].

### Awareness through Movement

A class setting is usually followed, and verbal instructions are given for movements, which lead to a heightened sensory awareness of the whole body. Learning through sensory experience, improved body alignment and mechanics are recognized and superfluous exertion eliminated.

### Functional Integration

This is based on the same principles that have been outlined above but is taught on an individual basis, with tactile feedback replacing verbal instructions. The subject's attention is drawn to the parts touched and, as the teacher moves these parts, to the connections between different parts of the body.

## 5.5.3. Pilates

Pilates is an exercise system that supports the vertebral column and activates and balances the trunk's postural muscles. It increases the awareness of vertebral columns' neutral position and strengthens the deep postural muscles. It emphasizes the mental concentration and spinal stabilization for muscle control and movement alignment. In the Pilates approach, it is a column that comprises the diaphragm in the top side, transversus abdominus in laterals, pelvic floor muscles in lower side and the multifudus muscle in back side. In all movements, the aim is to protect the central column and to continue during the movement. It also provides body awareness and activates body segments isolated [15,16,17,18,19,20].

During the exercises, head, neck, shoulders, and chest are positioned appropriately within the central column and combined with respiration. All steps of the motion must be integrated the body and mind. Because of this, it has limited usage for the patient with has low cognition.

In an MS patient, Pilates is useful for increasing body awareness, pelvis stabilization, and trunk control. Energy consumption should be decreased by Pilates.

Occasionally, techniques mentioned above may have unexpected side effects on spastic patients. These side effects occur due to excessive effort spent by a patient while trying to put body parts in desired positions and result in the aggravation of spasticity. Therefore, a patient should be observed closely during such exercises, and unnecessary muscular effort should be minimalized. If a patient continues to spend excessive effort, application should be discontinued.

## 5.6. CONCLUSION

Posture and gravity have mutual effects of a complex nature. Postural defects may be initialized by muscle weakness, muscle shortness or spasticity. Bad posture consequential of any of the factors above will aggravate the same factor as well. A postural problem starting from a specific body segment does not remain in that initial area; gradually the defect affects other body segments in a chain reaction.

Postural defects have negative outcomes not only on muscles and joints but also on joint ligaments, nervous system and lungs. Therefore, in physical therapy programmes, posture should be assessed profoundly and defects should be corrected in accordance with mechanical principles. Postural training should be initialized from pelvis, whether the training is actively performed by the patient or passively by the help of physiotherapist.

## 5.7. REFERENCES

[1]    Whitman, A. (1924). Postural deformities in children. *New York State Journal of Medicine* 2, 871-874

[2]    Pope, P.M. (1996). Postural management and special seating Chapter 7. İn Edwards, S. (eds.), *Neurological Physiotherapy: a problem-solving approach.* (eds 1) New York : Churchill Livingstone.

[3]    Kendall, H.O. & Kendall, F.P. & Boynton, D.A. (1952). *Posture and Pain,* Baltimore: Williams and Wilkins

[4]    Joseph, J. (1960). *Man's Posture.* Illinois: Charles C Thomas.

[5]    Woodhull, A.M. & Maltrud, K. & Mello, B.L. (1985). Alignment of the human body in standing. *European Journal of Applied Physiology,* 54, 109-115.

[6]    Jones, K. & Barker, K. (1996). *Human Movement Explained: Posture. Chapter 14.* (eds 12). Oxford: Butterworth and Heinemann.

[7]    Bullock-Saxton, J.E. (1993). Postural alignment in standing: a repeatability study. *Australian Journal of Physiotherapy,* 39, 25-29.

[8]   Baeppler, A. &, Kitkat, A. (1987). The Alexander technique. *Prof Nurse*
      2(7), 222-224.
[9]   Dennis, R.J. (1999). Functional reach improvement in normal older women
      after Alexander Technique instruction. *J Gerontol A Biol Sci Med Sci*,
      54(1), 8-11.
[10]  Stallibrass, C. & Sissons, P. & Chalmers, C. (2002). Randomized controlled
      trial of the Alexander technique for idiopathic Parkinson's disease. *Clin
      Rehabil*, 16(7), 695-708.
[11]  Ernst, E. & Canter, P.H. (2003). The Alexander technique: a systematic
      review of controlled clinical trials. *Forsch Komplementarmed Klass
      Naturheilkd*, 10(6), 325-9. Review.
[12]  [No authors listed]  (2008). Alexander technique helps relieve chronic back
      pain. *Harv Women's Health Watch*, 16(4), 7.
[13]  Feldenkrais, M. (1975). *Awareness Through Movement*, London: Penguin.
[14]  Santoro, F. & Maiorana, C.& Faccin, C. (1989). Neuromuscular relaxation
      and   CCMDP.   The   Zilgrei   and   Feldenkrais   methods   2   *Dent
      Cadmos*.31;57(16),  84-7
[15]  Blum, C.L (2002). Chiropractic and pilates therapy for the treatment of
      adult scoliosis. *J Manipulative Physiol Ther*, 25(4), 3.
[16]  Segal, N.A. & Hein, J. & Basford, J.R. (2004). The effects of Pilates
      training on flexibility and body composition: an observational study. *Arch
      Phys Med Rehabil*, 85(12), 1977-81.
[17]  Rydeard, R. & Leger, A. & Smith, D. (2006). Pilates-based therapeutic
      exercise: effect on subjects with nonspecific chronic low back pain and
      functional disability: a randomized controlled trial. *J Orthop Sports Phys
      Ther*, 36(7),472-84.
[18]  Curnow, D. & Cobbin, D. & Wyndham, J. & Boris Choy, S.T. (2009).
      Altered motor control, posture and the Pilates method of exercise
      prescription. *J Body Mov Ther*, 13(1), 104-11.
[19]  Kuo, Y.L. & Tully. E.A.& Galea. M.P. (2009). Sagittal spinal posture after
      Pilates-based exercise in healthy older adults. *Spine* 1;34(10), 1046-51.
[20]  Geweniger, V. (2002). Prevention of back pain with Pilates training: finding
      a healthy balance *Pflege Z*, 55(10), 747-9.

In: Spasticity and Its Management …       ISBN: 978-1-60876-185-5
Editor: Kadriye Armutlu       © 2010 Nova Science Publishers, Inc.

*Chapter 6*

# NEUROPHYSIOLOGICAL BASIS OF FACILITATION AND INHIBITION TECHNIQUES

## *Kadriye Armutlu*[*]

Hacettepe University, Faculty of Health Sciences, Department of Physical
Therapy and Rehabilitation, Neurological Rehabilitation Unit
06100/Ankara/TURKEY

## 6.1. ABSTRACT

Almost all physiotherapy applications are based on the principle of
facilitation or inhibition of proprioceptive and cutaneous senses, by way of
using appropriate techniques, which consequently results in the regulation of
motor outputs. Stimulating proprioceptors, mechanoceptors and cutaneal
receptors are used as a treatment in neurophysiologica-based physiotherapy.
There are special stimulating techniques for every kind of receptor. Although
proprioceptors and mechanoceptors have slow adaptation to a stimulus,
cuteneal receptors have fast adaptation a stimulus. As a result, it is
considered as a disadvantage for clinical applications.

Skeletal muscles have three main types of fibers, and these fibers have
different metabolic, mechanic and morphologic features. These are fast
twitch glycolytic fibers, fast twitch oxidative glycolytic fibers and slow
oxidative fibers. While planning the treatment, muscle fiber types should be
considered.

---

[*] Email: karmutlu@hacettepe.edu.tr

Key words: Facilitation and inhibition techniques, proprioceptive system, muscle spindle, golgi tendon organ, joint receptors. types of muscle fibers.

## 6.2. INTRODUCTION

Almost all physiotherapy applications are based on the principle of facilitation or inhibition of proprioceptive and cutaneous senses, by way of using appropriate techniques, which consequently results in the regulation motor outputs. Therefore, physical therapy applications are defined as approaches of neurophysiological basis.

Although the sensory system is the initiative means of inhibition and/or facilitation; muscle structures generating the motor output and their stimulation is important for the physiotherapist as well. Stimulation and inhibition of muscles depend on their fiber type and their covering area on joints (uni articular or bi articular).

This chapter is designed as a review of the propriocetive and cutaneous senses receptors, muscle types and stimulation forms in order to remind the physical therapist of the neurophysiological properties of the muscle and sensory system and probable reactions of the body during the application of techniques within the exercise programme.

## 6.3. PROPRIOCEPTIVE SYSTEM AND PROPER STIMULUS

The proprioceptive system is a complex structure consisting of muscle spindle (which is sensitive to muscle length), golgi tendon organ (sensitive to muscle tonicity) and mechanoreceptors. Each receptor has a different form of stimulation and response. Proprioceptors' adaptation to stimulus takes long time and is low [1, 2, 3, 4, 5]. Excitability level of receptors may differ as well. For instance, muscle spindle responds to stimulant rapidly, whereas summation may be required for the stimulation of golgi tendon organ. Receptors, stimulus and their responses are listed Tables 1 and 2 [6, 7, 8].

**Table 1. Muscle spindle**

| Receptor | Stimulus | Response |
| --- | --- | --- |
| Group Ia tonic | Length | Monosynaptic and polysynaptic facilitation of agonist muscle, polysynaptic inhibition of antagonist |
| Group Ia phasic | Rate of change in length | Monosynaptic facilitation of agonist muscle (stretch reflex), polysynaptic inhibition of antagonist |
| Group II | Length | Monosynaptic facilitation of agonist muscle (flexors), monosynaptic inhibition of antagonist (extensors) |

## Proper Facilitation Alternatives

- Quick stretch to agonist
- Tapping: the area near the motor point of the muscle
- Short-term cold application
- Positioning
- Stretch pressure
- Vibration within a facilitory frequency [9,10,11]
- Electrical stimulation

## Proper Facilitation Alternatives

- Maximal muscle contraction against resistance
- Tendon gripping or pressurizing
- Long-term stretch and passive positioning in extreme lengthened range

- Small, repeated contractions with gravity eliminated
- Manuel traction
- Manuel approximation [9, 10, 11, 12, 13, 14, 15, 16].

**Table 2. Golgi tendon organ and joint receptors**

| Receptor | Stimulus | Response |
|----------|----------|----------|
| Group Ib | Tension of tendon | Polysynaptic inhibition of agonist, facilitation of antagonist |
| *Joint receptors* | | |
| Group I | Static and dynamic joint tension: muscle pull | Stabilization of postural facilitation and joint position sense |
| Group II | Dynamic: rapid traction | Facilitation of agonist and joint position sense |
| Group III | Static: approximation | Agonist and antagonist co-contraction and stabilization |
| Group IV | Pain | Inhibition of agonist |

## Proper Facilitation Alternatives

- Painful stimulus: frequent use of  stimulating  flexor withdrawal reflex
- Short-duration cold application
- Light touch with finger tips or with a brush
- Fast stroking
- Vibration [17,18]

## 6.4. CUTANEOUS SYSTEM AND PROPER STIMULUS

### Table 3. Cutaneous Sense Receptors

| Receptors | Stimulus | Response |
|---|---|---|
| Free nerve endings: C and A fibers | Pain, temperature, touch | Facilitation of muscles under the related dermatome |
| Hair follicles | Mechanical displacement of hair receptors | Increase tone muscle under dermatome |
| Merkel's disk | Touch, pressure | Increase tone muscle under dermatome |
| Pacinian corpuscles | Deep pressure, rapid tension of the skin and vibration | Position sense, postural tone and increase tone muscle under dermatome |
| Ruffini's corpuscles | Touch mechanoreceptor | Increase tone muscle under dermatome |

**ATTENTION!**
Cutaneous sense receptors adapt rapidly, therefore, stimulations must not be applied successively.

# 6.5. TYPES OF MUSCLE FIBER AND PHYSIOLOGICAL FEATURES

Skeletal muscles have three main types of fibers, and these fibers have different metabolic, mechanic and morphologic features. Although each researcher has a different classification, the most commonly used form is as such [19, 20]:

- Fast twitch glycolytic (type II) (white) fibers
- Fast twitch oxidative glycolytic (type IIa) fibers
- Slow oxidative (type I) (red) fibers

Every muscle consists of these three fibers; however, density of the fiber varies according to the individual function of the muscle. If the rate of fast glycolytic fibers (type II) is high, the muscle is defined as "phasic." Phasic muscles twitch fast and tire rapidly, such as the hamstring group muscle activation during walking.

Slow oxidative (type I) type has endurance, twitches slowly and does not tire for long durations. These muscles are called tonic or stabilizing muscles. Antigravite muscles belong to this group.

If the fast oxidative glycolytic rate is high, the muscle is of intermediate characteristic.

Most muscles are formed from the combination of these fiber types. For instance: fast and slow twitch rates are almost equal in gastronecmius and deltoid muscles, whereas slow oxidative fiber rate is twice the rate of fast twitch in gastrosoleus. Basic differences between muscle fiber types are summed up in Table 4.

**Table 4. Characteristics of muscle fibers**

|  | Slow oxidative | Fast glycolytic | Fast oxidative glycolytic |
|---|---|---|---|
| *Color* | Red | White | Red |
| *Diameter* | Small | Large | Intermediate |
| *Speed of contraction* | Slow | Fast | Fast |
| *Rate of fatigue* | Slow | Fast | Intermediate |
| *Rate of recovery* | Fast | Slow | Intermediate |
| *Motor unit size* | Small | Large | Intermediate |

## 6.5.1. Treatment Principles According to Muscle Types

The body is a gross structure consisting of various types of muscles. People function differently in daily life depending on the distribution of muscle types. For instance, some people weary quickly whereas some are more enduring. These features are of major importance for athletes. They exercise proper sports in accordance with their body and muscle-fiber type (i.e., some run marathons and some are suitable for a 100m run). Muscle fiber type has a peculiar characteristic, which is the sensitivity for/towards training and immobilization. Characteristics of a fiber may alter due to training [21, 22]. Moreover, in cases of immobilization or neurological deficit-related spasticity, slow oxidative (type1) type fibers develop a fast glycolytic character resulting in fast weariness.

On this account, a survey of signs of clinical weakness and review of treatment principles will be beneficial for the physiotherapist [23, 24, 25].

*TONIC (POSTURAL) MUSCLES*
*Clinical signs of weakness:*
- Resting length changes, causing the muscle to lengthen
- Inability to maintain or hold a position against gravity
- Inability to hold a position in the shortest range
- Comes out abruptly from the stretch position
- Unilateral or asymmetrical holding (using movement muscles asymmetrically)
- Eccentric action is poor and collapses towards the end of the range.
- *Principal of treatment:*
- Align the part with postural muscles in the short range
- Use of sequence of activity in this order
  - o Isometric in the shortest possible range
  - o Eccentric in short range first and then controlled without collapse
  - o Concentric action as an exercise is done last or not at all
- Avoid long ranges until the muscle strengthens
- Progress from low-load resistance to higher loads

*PHASIC (MOVEMENT) MUSCLES*
*Principles of treatment of weak muscles:*
- Start in lengthened, but not extreme. Elongation is necessary to attain full shortening

- Strengthen by using isotonic shortening contractions through full range movement
- When using resistance, movement must be allowed
- Alternating active movements can be used
- Use tactile stimulation for facilitation
- Stiffness of antagonist muscles can be relieved by passive movements.

## 6.6. CONCLUSION

Neurophysiological physiotherapy methods are based on the principle of stimulation of numerous receptors as a means of treatment and using the responses derived from stimulation for the facilitation or inhibition of movement. The principle that antagonist of the facilitated muscle will be inhibited in return should be kept in mind. Each receptor has a specific stimulus and response.

Proprioceptors and mechanoreceptors adapt to stimulus at minimal, whereas cutaneous receptors' adaptation is fast and high; this difference is disadvantageous in terms of physical therapy applications. If the therapist is aiming at facilitation via stimulation of receptors, he must keep in mind that he may achieve desired responses only during the application of first few stimuli. Application of successive stimulants will have minimal effect on receptors.

Knowing the properties of muscle fibers will determine the course of treatment prescription. The therapist should keep the two principles in mind: weak tonic muscles should be strengthened within a short range; and strengthening of weak phasic muscle should be initiated by placing the muscle in a stretched position.

## 6.7. REFERENCES

[1]  Smith, J.L. & Crawford, M & Proske. U. & Taylor, J.L. (2009). Gandevia SC. Signals of motor command bias joint position sense in the presence of feedback from proprioceptors. *J Appl Physiol,* 106(3), 950-8

[2]  Stecco, C. & Gagey, O. (2007). Belloni A, Pozzuoli A, Porzionato A, Macchi V, Aldegheri R, De Caro R, Delmas V. Anatomy of the deep fascia of the upper limb. Second part: study of innervation. *Morphologie,* 91(292), 38-43.

[3]  Knikou, M. (2006). Effects of changes in hip position on actions of spinal inhibitory interneurons in humans. *Int J Neurosci,* 116(8), 945-61.

[4]  Sung, P.S. & Kang, Y.M. & Pickar. J.G. (2005). Effect of spinal manipulation duration on low threshold mechanoreceptors in lumbar paraspinal muscles: a preliminary report. *Spine,* 1;30(1), 115-22.

[5]  Lam, T. & Pearson K.G. (2002). The role of proprioceptive feedback in the regulation and adaptation of locomotor activity. *Adv Exp Med Biol.* 508, 343-55. Review.

[6]  Umphred D, Byl, N. & Lazaro, R. ( 2001). Interventions for Neurological Disabilities chapter 4. In Umphred DA (eds), *Neurological Rehabilitation.* (4. Edition). St. Louis: Mosby Company

[7]  Maurer, C. & Mergner, T. & Peterka, R.J. (2006). Multisensory control of human upright stance. *Exp Brain Res,* 171(2), 231-50.

[8]  Fromm, C. & Noth, J. & Thilmann, A. (1976). Inhibition of extensor gamma motoneurons by antagonistic primary and secondary spindle afferents. *Pflugers Arch.* 6;363(1), 81-6.

[9]  Roll, J.P. & Vedel, J.P. & Ribot, E. (1989). Alteration of proprioceptive messages induced by tendon vibration in man: a microneurographic study. *Exp Brain Res,* 76(1), 213-22.

[10] Montant, M. & Romaiguère, P. & Roll, J.P. (2009). A new vibrator to stimulate muscle proprioceptors in fMRI. *Hum Brain Mapp,* 30(3),990-7.

[11] Dyhre-Poulsen, P. & Krogsgaard, M.R. (2000). Muscular reflexes elicited by electrical stimulation of the anterior cruciate ligament in humans. *J Appl Physiol,* 89(6), 2191-5.

[12] Moraes, M.R. & Cavalcante, M.L. & Leite, J.A.& Ferreira, F.V. & Castro, A.J. & Santana, M.G. (2008) .Histomorphometric evaluation of mechanoreceptors and free nerve endings in human lateral ankle ligaments. *Foot Ankle Int,* 29(1),87-90.

[13] Armstrong, B. & McNair, P. & Taylor, D. (2008). Head and neck position sense. *Sports Med,* 38(2),101-17. Review.

[14] Proske, U. (2006). Kinesthesia: the role of muscle receptors. *Muscle Nerve,* 34(5),545-58. Review.

[15] Morningstar, M.W.& Pettibon, B.R. & Schlappi, H. & Schlappi, M. & Ireland, T.V. (2005). Reflex control of the spine and posture: a review of the literature from a chiropractic perspective. *Chiropr Osteopat,* 9,13:16.

[16] Macefield, V.G. (2005). Physiological characteristics of low-threshold mechanoreceptors in joints, muscle and skin in human subjects. *Clin Exp Pharmacol Physiol,* 32(1-2),135-44.

[17] Edin, B. (2001). Cutaneous afferents provide information about knee joint movements in humans. *J Physiol,* 15;531(Pt 1), 289-97.

[18] Brooke, J.D. & McIlroy, W.E. & Staines, W.R. & Angerilli, P.A. & Peritore G.F. (1999). Cutaneous reflexes of the human leg during passive movement. *J Physiol,* 15;518 (Pt 2),619-28.

[19] Huber, K. & Petzold, J. & Rehfeldt, C. & Ender, K. & Fiedler, I. (2007). Muscle energy metabolism: structural and functional features in different types of porcine striated muscles. *J Muscle Res Cell Motil,*28(4-5),249-58

[20] Jones, K. & Barker, K. (1996). *Human Movement Explained. Musculoskeletal basis of movement. Chapter 3.* (edition 12). Oxford: Butterworth and Heinemann.

[21] Thompson, L.V. (2002). Skeletal muscle adaptations with age, inactivity, and therapeutic exercise. *J Orthop Sports Phys Ther,* 32(2),44-57.

[22] Dupont-Versteegden, E.E. & Houlé, J.D. & Gurley, C.M. & Peterson, C.A. (1998). Early changes in muscle fiber size and gene expression in response to spinal cord transection and exercise. *Am J Physiol,* 275(4 Pt 1), 1124-1133.

[23] Stockmeyer, S.A. (1967). An interpretation of the approach of Rood to the treatment of neuromuscular dysfunction. *Am J Phys Med,* 46(1),900-961.

[24] Panturin, E. (1996). Hypotonic abdominal muscle in stroke patients. *Physiother Res Int,*1(4),269.

[25] Panturin, E. (2007). International Bobath Instructors Association Course Notes.

In: Spasticity and Its Management ...
Editor: Kadriye Armutlu

ISBN: 978-1-60876-185-5
© 2010 Nova Science Publishers, Inc.

*Chapter 7*

# EVALUATION OF THE PATIENT AND MEASUREMENT OF SPASTICITY

## *Kadriye Armutlu* * *and Yeliz Özçelik*

Hacettepe University, Faculty of Health Sciences, Department of Physical
Therapy and Rehabilitation, Neurological Rehabilitation Unit
06100/Ankara/TURKEY

## 7.1. ABSTRACT

When spasticity's high incidence, its negative effects and the subsequent costs for health care are considered, it is obvious that there is a profound need for accurate evaluation and quantification of spasticity. In order to choose the right technique among several, it is vital to detect the objective of assessment and define the aspects of spasticity needed to be evaluated. Assessment of a spastic patient should be initiated with anamnesis and observation. Muscle test, deep tendon reflexes, pathological reflexes and the measurement of passive and active ROM are important components in the process of evaluating spasticity. There are three primary techniques used for the quantitative measurement of spasticity (clinical scales, neurophysiological and biomechanical evaluations); but when a thorough evaluation is required, secondary measurement techniques may be of use alongside with primary ones. Despite their crucial limitations, both AS and MAS are still regarded as "golden standards" and widely preferred by clinicians for a clinical scale. Stretching reflex, tendon taps reflex (T reflex)

* Email: karmutlu@hacettepe.edu.tr

and Hoffmann reflex (H reflex) take place in neurophysiological evaluation, and they are important reflexes exposing the increased EMG response in spastic patient's pendulum test and isokinetic dynamometer. They are quite reliable methods, but because of their unfunctional application, they are not widely used in clinics. EDSS, Barthel index, Functional Independence Measurement, Functional Assessment Measurement, quality of life tests (i.e., SF-36, Nottingham Health Profile) are secondary measurements to be used alongside with primary ones.

Key words: Spasticity assessment, clinical scales, biomechanical techniques, neurophysiological techniques.

## 7.2. INTRODUCTON

Although the incidence of spasticity is not exactly known, it is assumed that over half a million people in the United States and 12 million people all over the world are subject to spasticity [1]. When spasticity's high incidence, its negative effects and the subsequent costs for health care are considered, it is obvious that there is a profound need for accurate evaluation and quantification of spasticity. An accurate evaluation of spasticity is fundamental for the determination of prognosis and assessment of efficient therapeutic, medical, surgical approaches of spasticity. Selection of the most efficient and cost-effective approach is only possible through an accurate evaluation and measurement.

Although there are several relatively reliable and patient-oriented measurement techniques, there is still not a specific technique valid for most cases. In order to choose the right technique among several, it is vital to detect the objective of assessment and define the aspects of spasticity that need to be evaluated.

The physiotherapist should follow the checklist below:

## 7.3. EXAMINATION OF A SPASTIC PATIENT

The physiotherapist's assessment starts at the moment of his/her first meeting with the patient. The patient's general body posture, walking pattern, presence of associated reactions and his walking support provide the initial information that guides the physical therapist in determining the evaluation and measurement methods.

| Evaluation and measurement checklist |
|---|
| ❖ *Meeting with the patient and patient acquaintance, surveying the file consisting of personal and medical data about the patient.*<br>✓ First impression about general physical appearance of the patient, observing his walk and other movements<br>✓ Determining/verifying specific difficulties encountered by the patient during his daily life activities, caused by MS in general and spasticity in particular, based on the patient's own statements.<br>✓ Review of medical treatments and medication being applied.<br>✓ Questioning bladder problems, self-catheterization and urinary tract infections<br>❖ *Physical Examination*<br>✓ Examination of the skin and fingernails; palpation of other soft tissues<br>✓ Posture analysis<br>✓ Examining alterations in muscle tone in different body positions<br>✓ Determining the effect of effort on muscle tone<br>✓ Analysis of pathological responses<br>✓ Application of strength test on antispastic muscles and, if necessary, on spastic muscles as well.<br>✓ Measurement of active and passive joint range of motion and application of muscle length tests<br>✓ Evaluation of superficial sense and position sense<br>✓ Ataxia and balance tests<br>✓ Evaluation of fatigue<br>✓ Use of supplementary scales and/or methods designed for the measurement of spasticity<br>✓ Determination of phase of the disease<br>✓ Making the treatment prescription and determining the treatment objectives in accordance with evaluation and assessment findings<br>✓ Informing the patient and patient's relatives about the treatment plan |

Assessment of a spastic patient should be initiated with anamnesis and observation. The physical therapist then uses the attained information to find out how the patient's current functionality, quality of life and everyday activities are affected, relying on the patient's personal experiences. Following the transcription of case history, the effect of spasticity on the patient's functional and daily life activities should be observed closely. For instance, hip adduction and flexion spasticity complicates hygiene and dressing. However, it should be kept in mind that spasticity may be advantageous while performing some activities: for example, an increase in extensory tonus in the lower extremity may have positive effects during the transfer and ambulation of the patient. Therefore, the detrimental and beneficial effects of spasticity should be clarified through observation [2,3,].

Subsequently, the physical therapist should make his own personal file of the patient, covering data about his medication—corticosteroids in particular—and dosage of medication at present by use of patient's formal medical records and his personal statements. If the patient has been or is on corticosteroids, bone densimetry findings should be surveyed by the physical therapist. Specifically, if an a osteoporothic situation is observed, concerning the femoris corpus or collum and lumbar vertebras, the physical therapist should be sensitive in making the exercise prescription because of the high risk of fractures.

Usage of interferons should also be taken into consideration since it is fundamental in means of spasticity. Type and usage frequency and skin reactions related to interferons should be noted. Apart from these applications, the patient should be questioned about the antispastic medication used, beneficial aspects of the medicaments, and if he had suffered from the side-effects such as sedation, fatigue, balance deficits, etc. If the patient has excessive complaints about the side-effects, the physical therapist should get in touch with the related specialist to adjust dosage. The physiotherapist should also be informed if botilinum toxin is applied in order to manage spasticity, the muscle groups it was applied on and frequency of application.

During the meeting with the patient, bladder problems, frequency of urinary tract infections and exercise of self-catheterization should be surveyed.

During the examination, the patient should be asked whether he has flexor spasms; and if so, the frequency and localization of the spasms are to be inquired. Furthermore, it is important to question and determine the factors of aggravated flexor spasms.

Factors that may have negative effects on flexor spasms and spasticity should be determined through palpation and observation. During the examination, the patient is asked to undress, just leaving the underwear on, in order to observe the skin closely and palpate the stiff areas. Toenails, in particular, should be examined to find out if there are nail immersions, and, if so, the patient should be directed to the related specialist.

Furthermore, it should be clarified if spasticity, sensed by the patient himself, is increasing depending on posture, different positions, effort and emotional changes.

Increase in muscle tonicity has negative effects on the skeleto-muscular system and posture. Therefore, posture should be examined in detail and alterations should be transcribed (i.e., retractions in pelvis and shoulders, inversion in ankles…). In addition, alterations in the points of gravity line of the patient should be observed. For instance, if the patient has developed an anterior balance, the gravity line would glide forward. Or, the patient may have developed a balance by leaning towards right or left. In such a case under suspect, "plumb-line test," which is the simplest method of assessment in clinical practice, should be used. This test is applied laterally and posteriorly, through which it is observed whether the plumb passes from the points of reference, and variances are noted down in centimeters. Patients with anterior balance, in particular, should be perturbated towards the posterior by the physiotherapist, and their responses to the movement should be observed closely (i.e., sudden giving way of the knee indicates that quadriceps femoris does not have sufficient strength). In some clinics, posturography devices are frequently used; if there are such means, alterations of gravity center within the support surface may be measured by computer.

Since it would be misleading to evaluate spasticity with a single (bodily) position, the patient should be examined in several different postures as well. When a good case history is attained, statements of the patient about his complaints will be clear enough to support the case history itself. For example: if a patient's spasticity is increasing in accordance with gravity; he will state that he feels as if his feet are stuck to the ground when he stands up or he has difficulties bending his knees. Or, if the patient has a spasticity increasing with effort, he will convey that he feels stiffness in his legs while walking.

Moreover, pathological responses, such as positive support reaction, flexor withdrawal response, grasping reflex, clonus and associated reactions, should be filtered thoroughly and their negative effects on the posture should be taken into consideration. For instance, positive support reaction is a static response of lower extremity, occurring when the foot touches the ground (pressure stimulus). Both antagonist and agonist muscle groups are affected and an increase in extensor tonicity of lower extremity occurs (figure 1). In order to keep in poise and neutralize these effects, some compensatory strategies like pelvis retraction and body flexion develop. As a result of pelvis retraction, hip flexor adductors and medial rotators shrink. Another consequence of this reaction is tibialis posterior spasticity, which results in ankle inversion and plantar flexion, shrinking of intrinsic foot muscle and range loss in plantar fasia (figure 2). The treatment programme should be managed depending on the findings of an extensive assessment of so-mentioned alterations [4]

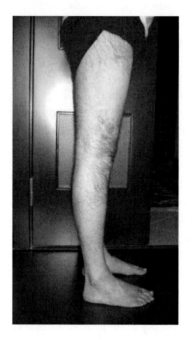

Figure 1. Positive support reaction.

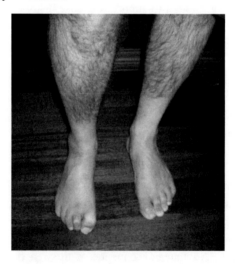

Figure 2. Intrinsic foot muscle spasticity.

Achilles clonus (a pathological reflex) is of functional importance for physiotherapists. Clonus is generated by the sudden stretching of plantar flexors, and it may result in imbalance while standing up or cause problems in hitting the gas/break pedals while driving.

Muscle test, deep tendon reflexes, clonus and the measurement of passive and active ROM are important components in the process of evaluating spasticity [5].

In most cases of spasticity, loss of strength in muscles constitutes the major factor causing disability. Formerly, conducting muscle strength test to the spastic muscle was avoided. However, on the basis of current findings, it is known that in a spastic muscle, type II muscle fibers are transformed into type I and generate atrophy in the fibers of type II muscle [4]. Therefore, it would be misleading to assume that a spastic muscle is always strong. Spastic muscle may be strong in a sinergistic pattern but when the muscle is taken out of this pattern and normal motion is forced to facilitate, the muscle weakens. This outcome forms the basis of quite a few neurological approaches that argue the necessity of replacement of sinergistic patterns with normal motion patterns. Although it is not possible to conduct muscle strength test when synergistic patterns and associated reactions are present, the test should be applied to every single muscle that is able to perform an isolated joint motion. Evaluation of muscle strength in a spastic patient is also important for the selection of the appropriate orthesis. For instance, when a decision is made to splint an ankle with plantar flexion spasticity, the strength of spastic quadriceps femoris should be taken into consideration. Despite being spastic, this muscle may not have the necessary strength. As a result of the usage of orthesis, flexion moment may fade in, weakening the knees and causing difficulties in standing up.

Spasticity may limit active and passive ROM by causing biomechanical alterations primarily in muscle structure and secondarily in joint structure. Therefore, it is important to determine active and passive joint motion limitation accurately. Goniometer, which is a simple and clinically functional device, may be preferred. Although it is difficult for spastic patients to pose for goniometric measurement, by making custom adaptations, every joint can be measured [6].

Analysis of clasp knife phenomenon and velocity dependent component of spasticity is fundamental in distinguishing neural component of spasticity from non-neural component. As spasticity grows chronic, its dependence on velocity decreases, followed by a gradual decline and discontinuation of clasp knife phenomenon. These are signs of alterations in the intrinsic structure of the muscle marking the recent dominance of non-neural component of spasticity. Awareness of these alterations will guide the physiotherapist through making the physical treatment prescription considering the use of manual techniques and orthoses.

**ATTENTION!**
Patient cannot benefit from botilinum toxin application if his spasticity has developed non-neural component.

Presence of sensory problems affects therapist's choice of antispastic applications. Loss/declining of senses of touch, vibration, temperatures, movement and position is highly common among MS patients [7]. Superficial senses of temperature, superficial pain and touch are particularly important for the physical therapist. Cold/hot sticks, a cotton ball or a pin may be used as test materials. The test should cover the fundamental dermatomes (i.e., leg, arm, hand and forearm are more important for the physiotherapist than the other parts of the body). Findings should be marked on a dermatome card.

Among the proprioceptive senses, particularly the position and movement sense should be assessed. Sensation of motion and position may also be tested by placing the fingers of one of the **patient's hands** in a specific position while his eyes are closed, then asking him to describe the position or to imitate it with the other hand. The foot may be passively moved while eyes are closed, and the patient is asked his foot position [8].The same procedure may be applied to the first three toes. The knee is as of equal importance as the ankle in the management of lower extremity movement. The mechanical integrity of foot, knee and hips should all be considered for the management of spasticity in MS patients. Comparative tests should be applied both to upper and lower extremities.

MS differs from other CVA diseases that have spasticity as a major symptom, in terms of spasticity being accompanied by ataxia. The type walk of MS patients is spastic ataxic. Imbalance during mobilization and unequal step/pace are usually the indicators of ataxia, which generates a complex outcome; since spasticity is sometimes managed by way of stabilizing the effects of ataxia and over-relaxing a spastic muscle during the process, it may lead to total imbalance or vice versa. Therefore, the therapist should analyze balance problems of the patient multidimensionally and define the effects of these problems on spasticity. In clinical practice, Berg Balance Scale is the most frequently used one, a reliable and valid scale for the evaluation of functional balance, particularly in MS patients.

Fatigue is an important parameter of assessment. The patient should be questioned if he has complaints of fatigue. If so, its formality and effects on functions should be inquired. The Fatigue Severity Scale is commonly used for the evaluation of fatigue [9]. Motor fatigue is another parameter of assessment. Motor fatigue in MS patients is usually evaluated by Walking Fatigue. This is actualized by recording the walking speed of patients in the first and last 50 m.s of 500 or 200m.s walks. Findings are placed in the formulation below:

V (velocity): walking distance/time
Walking fatigue index: 100%x [1-(V last 50m/V first 50m) [10].

The quantitative measurement of spasticity is quite difficult and complicated. It is dependent on the assessor's experiences. Findings may vary even within the same day, related to personal and environmental factors. Extremity and changes in posture during the evaluation process affect the intensity of spasticity. For instance, changes in head and neck postures while tonic labyrinth and tonic neck reflexes are active affect the severity of spasticity. Furthermore, increasing body or room temperature and intense fatigue also affect the severity of spasticity [3].

There are three primary techniques used for the quantitative measurement of spasticity (clinical scales, neurophysiological and biomechanical evaluations); but when a thorough evaluation is required, secondary measurement techniques may be of use alongside with primary ones [11, 12, 13].

**Primary Techniques**
Clinical scales
Biomechanical Assessment
    Pendulum Tests
    Isokinetic Dynamometer
Neurophysiological and Electrophysiological Assessment
    H Response
    H/M Ratio
    F Response, F/M Ratio
    Other Reflex Studies
**Secondary Techniques**
Gaite analysis
Activity of daily living tests
Quality of life tests

Nine-hole peg test, Perdue-peg board, Minnesota test for upper limb spasticity

## 7.4. PRIMARY TECHNIQUES

### 7.4.1. Clinical Scales

In clinical scales, severity of spasticity is assessed by a subjective measurement of resistance to passive movement. Limitation at this point is that resistance against passive movement is not only originated from the neural component of spasticity, but it is also affected by non-neural factors such as joint and soft tissue stiffness. Therefore, distinguishing the resistance originating from neural components from the resistance originating from soft tissue alterations is fundamental since they respond to different treatments. Another limitation of clinical scales is that due to its velocity-oriented nature, severity of spasticity is subject to changes related to the stretching velocity manipulated by the clinician. According to the findings of a number of studies, correlation between clinical scales is usually poor; they measure different aspects of spasticity and are deficient in measuring the differences between neural and non-neural components. Therefore, in order to obtain a comprehensive assessment, various scales are to be applied on a single patient [14-15].

#### *Ashworth and Modified Ashworth Scale*
Ashworth scale (AS) was developed in 1964, to assess drug efficiency in MS patients [16]. In this scale, muscle tonicity is rated between zero (normal) and four (severe spasticity). In 1987, Bohannon and Smith developed the Modified Ashworth Scale (MAS), by adding +1 score between scores one and two, to increase the sensitivity of the scale [17]. Although both scales are widely used in clinics, they measure not the velocity dependent reflex response of spasticity but its resistance to passive movement [18] (see appendix 1,2).

There are a number of studies on the reliability and validity of AS and MAS, but the findings of these studies are conflicting. Although studies made on several different patient groups at different times report that AS and MAS are reliable and valid scales [19,20], AS is more reliable on distal muscle groups and less reliable when proximal muscle groups are concerned [21]. According to another study comparing wrist flexors with knee extensors, MAS proved to be reliable for wrist spasticity and not reliable for knee extansors [22]. In fact, clinical assessments show that minimal spasticity in knee extansors is sensed at the beginning of the movement, whereas minimal resistance against passive movement is sensed at the end of the movement in other muscle groups.

Studies comparing the two scales show that their reliabilities are quite low and that there is no significant difference between the two [23]. Despite their crucial limitations, both AS and MAS are still regarded as "golden standards" and widely preferred by clinicians.

## Tardieu Scale

The scale is developed in 1954, by Tardieu et al. [24]. The most distinctive quality of Tardieu scale (TS) is its ability to expose the velocity dependent nature of spasticity by actualizing passive stretching in three different velocities. In 1999, Boyd and Graham developed Modified Tardieu Scale (MTS) by adding extremity measuring positions and spasticity angle to the original scale [25] (see appendix 3).

In a study concerning children with cerebral palsy, MAS, MTS and Wartenberg pendulum tests were compared and MTS turned out to be the most adequate technique  (MTS is generally preferred on children rather than adult patients in most cases) [26].

## Multiple Sclerosis Spasticity Scale

This scale, developed particularly for MS patients in 2006, by Hobart et al., not only measures symptoms of spasticity but also proves to be a valid and reliable assessment technique for inquiring about the effects of spasticity in patient's experiences and his quality of life. The scale consists of eight sections; three sections assess spasticity symptoms (muscle stiffness, pain, muscle spasms), three sections assess physical functions (walking, daily life activities, and body motions), one section assesses emotional condition and one section assesses social functions [27] (see appendix 4).

## Numeric Rating Scale

Numeric rating scale (NRS) is a verbal scale, demanding the measurement of spasticity by the patient himself, rating the intensity of spasticity on a scale of zero to ten. Studies assessing its reliability and validity were made on MS patients in 2008 [28]. A study comparing NRS with clinical assessments (MAS) detected a weak correlation between the two (Spearman p range 0.44 to 0.62) [29]. Despite this poor correlation, in the literature, it is stated that patients' own findings are as important as that of clinicians', in defining the severity of spasticity (see appendix 5).

*Spasm Frequency Scale-Penn Spasm Scale*

Spastic patients may have spasms affecting their functional activities and causing sleep disorders. Spasms are measured by recording the number of spontaneous muscle spasms occurring in a one-hour period. In the literature, Spasm Frequency Scale and Penn Spasm Scale are considered reliable and valid techniques designed for this measurement [30, 31] (see appendix 6,7).


## 7.4.2. Biomechanical Measurements

Biomechanical measurements are used for assessing the mechanical response of the muscle to a controlled stimulus. The assessment aims at measuring the severity of spasticity by detecting the correlation between torque (rotating moment) and angle following the controlled passive stretching. Price divided these techniques into four groups: manual, controlled displacement, controlled torque and gravitational methods [32]. In literature, generally the Wartenberg Pendulum test (which is a subcategory of gravitational methods) and isokinetic measurements (subcategory of controlled displacement) are more preferred than other techniques.


*Pendulum Test*

The Pendulum test was developed by Wartenberg in 1951, to measure the severity of spasticity. The test makes use of gravity in order to measure the spasticity in hamstring and quadriceps muscles [33]. It is widely used in literature and has recently been adapted for the measurement of elbow muscle spasticity [34.] During testing, the patient lies down or is seated, letting his legs hang down from the sides of the examination table. The patient's knee is held in a fully extended position for some time. When total relaxation is secured, the knee is released to swing freely. The pendulum-like movements of the knee are recorded by electrogoniometer and movement rate is recorded by tachometer. Decrease in oscillatory movements in spastic patients shows itself by decreased or faded sinusoid patterns in graphics. What needs to be kept in mind about the Pendulum test is that its findings vary depending both on spasticity and mechanical structure of patient's leg as well [3].


*Isokinetic Dynamometer*

Isokinetic dynamometer measures the severity of spasticity by its resistance against passive movement in a particular angle and velocity through calculating parameters like peak torque, torque and threshold angle. Studies on its reliability and validity were performed on several neurological patients, particularly on those with SCI. When spasticity's velocity dependent nature is considered, isokinetic dynamometer proved to be a quite reliable method. But because of its unfunctional application, it is not widely used in clinics [35 , 36 ].

## 7.4.3. Neurophysiological Measurements

The most commonly accepted method to measure spasticity is detecting abnormal muscle contractions by using multi-channel EMG. However, it should be considered that electrical signals derived from the relaxed muscles have no clinical significance and that distonia in spontaneous EMG activity makes it impossible to differentiate between spasm and spasticity. In order to determine spasticity, EMG signals generated particularly during the stretching reflex are to be sorted out. Stretching reflex, tendon taps reflex (T reflex) and Hoffmann reflex (H reflex) are important reflexes exposing the increased EMG response in spastic patients.

### *Hoffmann Reflex*
It was defined by Piper in 1912, and expanded by Hoffmann in 1918 [37]. Hoffmann reflex is a monosynaptic reflex obtained by the stimulation of posterior tibial nerve in posterior fossa, eliciting a reflex response in the triceps surae musle [38]. It precisely denotes the level of alfa motor neuron excitability. Although the latency of this reflex does not alter in spastic patients, its amplitude increases. When H reflex is inhibited by applying vibration to Achilles tendon, the outcome is called "tonic vibration reflex" [2 ].

### *H/M Ratio*
When stimulation given to the posterior tibial muscle nerve to develop H reflex is supramaximal, a reflex called M reflex generates in the same muscle. Since H/M ratio tends to be higher in spastic patients, during the assessment process, determination of M reflex is particularly important [39].

### *F Response - F/M Ratio*
F response has less amplitude and shorter latency than M reflex. It denotes alfa motor neuron excitability. There is an increase in F/M ratio in MS patients [2].

## 7.5. SECONDARY MEASUREMENTS

By using the gait analysis conducted through multi-channel EMG, different muscle groups in activation, power developed in lower extremity and joint angles can be studied altogether. Furthermore, important parameters of ambulation/gait (such as footpace, walking speed, cadence) are analyzed, and the rate of spasticity, effecting the movement is determined [40, 41].

Walking analysis does not require computerized systems by all means. The Footprint test, which is a simple method of clinical evaluation, may also be used. The patient walks on a powdered surface and his footprints are measured to determine support surface, step length and stride length (figure 3).

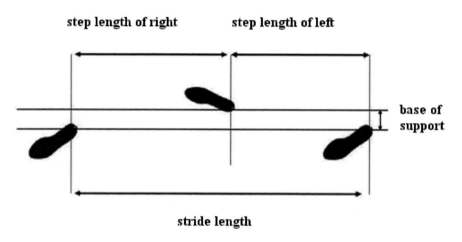

Figure 3. Gait analysis with footprint method.

EDSS, Barthel index, Functional Independence Measurement, Functional Assessment Measurement, quality of life tests (i.e., SF-36, Nottingham Health Profile) are secondary measurements to be used alongside with primary ones. To assess the upper extremity spasticity, functional tests such as Nine Peg Hold test, Perdue-Peg Board and Minnesota can be applied.

Although the quantitative measurement of spasticity is quite difficult, there are a number of studies and methods composed to ease the process. Experiences of the clinician are essential in selecting the most appropriate and reliable technique among many. When a comprehensive measurement introducing spasticity in every possible aspect is required, the most accurate approach would be using not one but several scales. In research studies, the usage of neurophysiological and biomechanical techniques along with clinical assessment scales will provide clinicians with more objective findings. Furthermore, it should be kept in mind that personal assessments of the patient are not to be considered as a subjective method but as an enlightening approach. As a consequence, the fact that there is no single valid scale for spastic measurement and that spasticity still has many uncovered aspects should be accepted for the time being.

The physiotherapist interprets the findings of evaluation and assessment and determines his treatment goals and antispastic applications according to the severity of spasticity, muscles affected by spasticity (focal of general), presence of muscle/joint contractures and sensory problems. Physical treatment prescription should be made in accordance with the complementary treatment principle by taking the secondary muscle weakness, fatigue, mobilization level and psychosocial state of the patient into consideration. For instance, some patients may refuse to use orthosis for aesthetic concerns. In such cases, the use of orthoses should be delayed for a while and the therapist should try to manage spasticity with alternative methods. In the advanced stages of treatment, the use of orthosis may come to the scene.

Efficiency of antispastic treatment varies from one patient to another and depends on the outcomes and phase of spasticity. The phase of the disease is indicated by scores of the patient on EDSS. The disease has four phases:

Phase 1: beginning (diagnostic phase) (EDSS minimum 1)
Phase 2: early phase (minimal disability) (EDSS 1 to 5.5)
Phase 3: middle phase (mediocre disability) (EDSS 6 to 7.0)
Phase 4: advanced phase (severe disability) (EDSS >7) [42].

The physical therapist aims at attaining a more symmetrical and neutral walking pattern for the patient with minimal and focal spasticity. Whereas the goal is to reduce energy consumption and increase walking distance in a patient with mediocre generalized spasticity, if the patient has drastically severe generalized spasticity, the therapist should focus on slowing down the development of contractures and maintaining a comfortable sitting/lying down position.

Success of neurological rehabilitation is bound to the consistency and communication between the patient (and his relatives) and the rehabilitation team. The patient constitutes the center of all applications. The physiotherapist should share the treatment plan and goals with the patient, inform him that the management of MS and spasticity may take quite a long time and make sure that the patient understands that the home-exercises are as important as the supervised ones. Spasticity demands a 24-hour encounter, which can only be managed if the patient himself, patient's relatives and the rehabilitation team work together in coordination.

## 7.6. CONCLUSION

Assessment of MS patients by taking spasticity and other symptoms into consideration is essential for the correct analysis of outcomes and determination of proper treatment programmes. Therefore, assessment and evaluations must be multi-dimensional.

There are a large number of scales and methods developed for the evaluation and assessment of spasticity. Use of these scales is advantageous, since findings attained are numerical. However, the scales are not sensitive to all characteristics and outcomes of MS, which makes them inadequate for a complete assessment of spasticity. Therefore, personal findings of the physiotherapist, obtained from observation, examination and by listening to the patient, are crucial for the assessment process as well. An experienced physiotherapist analyzes the findings, determines his goals and shares them with patient, the patient's relatives and the rehabilitation team. Well-documented assessment-evaluation findings play an important role in patient's responses to physical therapy and other treatments and monitoring progression of the disease.

## 7.7. REFERENCES

[1]    Vanek,    Z.    Spasticity.    (2007    Aug    29).    Available    from: www.emedicine.com/neuro/topic706. htm
[2]    Katz, R.T. & Dewald J.P.A & Schmit B.D. (2000). Spasticity. In Braddom R.L. (eds.), *Physical medicine and rehabilitation* (edition 2, pp 592-615). Philadelphia: W. B. Saunders Company.
[3]    Gelber, A. & Douglas, R.F. (2002). *Clinical evaluation and management of spasticity* (1 edition). Totowa, New Jersey: Humana Press.
[4]    Edward, S. (1996). *Neurological physiotherapy: a problem-solving approach* (edition 1). New York: Churchill Livingstone.
[5]    Skold, C. & Levi, R. & Seiger A. (1999). Spasticity after traumatic spinal cord injury: nature, severity, and location. *Arch Phys Med Rehabil*,80,1548-1557.

[6]     Stevenson, V.L. & Louise, J. (2006). *Spasticity management: a practical multidisciplinary guide* (edition 1). Oxon: İnforma Healthcare.

[7]     Osterberg, A & Boivie, J. & Thuomas KA. (2005).Central pain in multiple sclerosis—prevalence and clinical characteristics. *Eur J Pain.* 9(5):531-42. Epub 2004 Dec 22.

[8]     Haerer, A. F. (1992) *DeJong's the neurological examination.* (Edition 5). JB Lippincot Company: Philadelphia.

[9]     Krupp, L. B & LaRocca, N. G. Muir-Nash, J. & Steinberg, A. D (1989). Fatigue severity scale: aplication to patients with multiple sclerosis and systemic lupus erythematosus. *Arch Neurol,* 46, 1121-1123.

[10]    Schwid, S.R & Covington, M. & Segal, B.M. & Goodman, A.D. (2002). Fatigue in multiple sclerosis: current understanding and future directions. *J Rehabil Res Dev.*39 (2), 211-24.

[11]    Platz, T. & Eickhof, C. & Nuyens G. & Vuadens P. (2005). Clinical scales for the assessment of spasticity, associated phenomena, and function: a systematic review of the literature. *Disabil Rehabil,* 27, 7-18.

[12]    Wood, D.E. & Burrıdge, J.H. & Van Wıjck, F.M. & Mcfadden, C. & Hıtchcock, R.A. & Pandyan, A.D. & Haugh, A. & Salazar-Torres, J.J & Swaın, I.D. (2005). Biomechanical approaches applied to the lower and upper limb for the measurement of spasticity: A systematic review of the literature, *Disability and Rehabilitation,* 27(1/2), 19–32.

[13]    Voerman, G.E. & Gregorıc, M. & Hermens, H.J. (2005). Neurophysiological methods for the assessment of spasticity: The Hoffmann reflex, the tendon reflex, and the stretch reflex, *Disability and Rehabilitation,* 27(1/2), 33–68.

[14]    Priebe, M.M & Sherwood, A.M & Thornby, J.I & Kharas, N.F. & Markowski, J. (1996). Clinical assessment of spasticity in spinal cord injury: a multidimensional problem. *Arch Phys Med Rehabil,* 77, 713-716.

[15]    Pirotte, B. & Heilporn, A. & Joffroy, A. & Zegers de Beyl, D. & Wesel, P. & Brotchi, J. & Levivier M. (1996). Chronic intrathecal baclofen in several disabling spasticity, Selection clinical assessment and long-term benefit. *Acta Neurol Belg,* 4, 267–269.

[16]    Ashworth, B. (1964). Preliminary trial of carisoprodol in multiple sclerosis. *Practitioner,* 192, 540-542.

[17]    Bohannon, R.W. & Smith, M.B. (1987). Interrater reliability of a Modified Ashworth Scale of muscle spasticity. *Phys Ther,* 67, 206-207.

[18]    Andra Calota, A.B. & Anatol, G. & Feldman, B.C & Mindy F. & Levin, AB. (2008). Spasticity measurement based on tonic stretch reflex threshold in stroke using a portable device. *Clin Neurophysiol,* 119(10), 2329-2337.

[19] Lee, K. & Carson, L. & Kinine, E. & Patterson, V. (1989).The Ashwoth Scale: A reliable and reproducible method of measuring spasticity. *Journal Neurological Rehabilitation,* 3, 205- 209.

[20] Bohannon, R.W. & Smith, M.B. O (1987). Inter-rater reliability of a Modified Ashworth Scale of muscle spasticity. *Physiotherapy,* 67, 206-207.

[21] Nuyens, G. & De Weerdt, W. & Ketelaer, P. & Feys, H. & De Wolf L. & Hantson, L. & Nieuboer, A. & Spaepen, A. & Carton, H. & (1994). Inter-rater reliability of the Ashworth Scale in multiple sclerosis. *Clinical Rehabilitation,* 8, 286-292.

[22] Sloan, R.L. & Sinclair, E. & Thompson, J. & Taylor, S. & Pentland, B. (1992). Inter-rater reliability of the Modified Ashworth Scale for spasticity in hemiplegic patients. *International Journal Rehabilitation Research,* 15, 158-161.

[23] Hass, B.M. & Bergstrom, E. & Jamous, A. & Bennie, A. (1996). The inter-rater reliability of the original and of the Modified Ashworth Scale for the assessment of spasticity in patients with spinal cord injury. *Spinal Cord,* 34, 560-564.

[24] Tardieu, G. & Shentoub, S. & Delarue, R.A. (1954). La recherche d'une technique de measure de la spasticite. *Rev Neurol (Paris),* 91, 143–144.

[25] Boyd, R.N. & Graham, H.K. (1999). Objective measurement of clinical findings in the use of botulinum toxin type A for the management of children with cerebral palsy. *Eur J Neurol,* 6(Suppl. 4), S23–S35.

[26] Amman, C.M. & Kawanami, L.M. & Giratalla, M.M. & Hoetmer, R.A. & Rodriguez, V.J. & Munro, K.K. et al. (2005). Choosing a Spasticity Outcome Measure: A Review for the Neuromodulation Clinic. *UAHSJ,* 2, 29-32.

[27] Hobart,, J.C. & Riazi, A. & Thompson, A.J. & Styles, I.M. & Ingram, W. & Vickery, P.J. & Warner, M. & Fox, P.J. & Zajicek, J.P. (2006). Getting the measure of spasticity in Multiple Sclerosis: the Multiple Sclerosis Spasticity Scale (MSSS-88*). Brain,* 129, 224-34.

[28] Farrar, J.T. & Troxel, A.B. & Stott, C. & Duncombe, P. & Jensen, M.P. (2008) Validity, Reliability, and Clinical Importance of Change in a 0–10 Numeric Rating Scale Measure of Spasticity: A Post Hoc Analysis of a Randomized, Double-Blind, Placebo-Controlled Trial. *Clinical Therapeutics,* 30(5), 224-234.

[29] Skold, C. (2000). Spasticity in spinal cord injury: self- and clinically rated intrinsic fluctuations and intervention-induced changes. *Arch Phys Med Rehabil,* 81, 144-149.

[30] Penn, R.D. & Savoy, S.D. & Corcos, D. & Latash, M. & Gottlieb, G. & Parke, B., et al. (1989). Intrathecal baclofen for severe spasticity. *N Engl J Med*, 320, 1517-1521.

[31] Pedersen, E. & Klemar, B. & Torring, J. (1979). Counting of Flexor Spasm. *Acta Neural Scand*, 60, 164-169.

[32] Price, R. (1990). Mechanical spasticity evaluation techniques. *Critical Reviews in Physical Rehabilitation Medicine*, 2, 65–73.

[33] Wartenberg, R. (1951). Pendulousness of the leg as a diagnostic test. *Neurology*, 1, 18–24.

[34] Lin, C.C. & Ju, M.S. & Lin, C.W. (2003). The pendulum test for evaluation spasticity of the elbow joint. *Arch Phys Med Rehabil*, 84, 69–74.

[35] Boiteau, M. & Malouin, F. & Richards, C.L. (1995). Use of hand-held dynamometer and a KinComdynamometer for evaluating spastic hypertonia in children: a reliability study. *Phys Ther*, 75, 796–802.

[36] Akman, M.N. & Bengi, R. & Karatas, M.& Kilinc, S. & Sozay, S. & Ozker, R. (1999). Assessment of spasticity using isokinetic dynamometry in patients with spinal cord injury. *Spinal Cord*, 37(9), 638–643.

[37] Piper, H. (1912). Die Aktionsstro¨me menschlicher Muskeln. Die Metodiek der Untersuchung am Seitengalvanometer und die Prinzipien der Stromkurvenanalyse. Typennunterschiede der Willku¨ rkontraktion. Zeitung *Biol Tech Methode*, 3, 52.

[38] Fisher, M.A. (1992). AAEM Minimonograph #13: H reflexes and F waves: Physiology and clinical indications. *Muscle and Nerve*, 15, 1223–1233.

[39] Garrett, M. & Caulfield, B. (1996). Modulation of the Hoffmann reflex of soleus during the walking cycle in stroke patients and associated control of ankle joint movement. In Pedotti A. & Ferrarin M. & Quintern J. & Riener R. (eds.), *Neuroprosthetics. From basic research to clinical application* (pp. 51-58). Berlin Heidelberg: Springer–Verlag.

[40] Flipetti, P. & Decq, P. & Fontaine, D. & Feve, A. & Pirotte, A. & Barbedette, B. & et al. (1998). Lower limb spasticity in adults. Clinical evaluation with motor block. *Neurochirurgie*, 44,167-74.

[41] Fung, J. & Barbeau, H. (1989). A Dynamic Emg Profile İndex To Quantify Muscular Activation Disorder İn Spastic Paretic Gait. *Electroencephalogr Clin Neurophysiol*, 73, 233-234.

[42] Kurtzke, J.F. (1983). Rating neurologic impairment in multiple sclerosis: An expanded disability status scale (EDSS). *Neurology*, 33(11), 1444-1452.

# APPENDICIES

## APPENDIX 1

### Ashworth Scale

| Grade | Description |
|-------|-------------|
| 0 | No increase in tone |
| 1 | Slight increase in tone giving catch when the limb is moved in flexion and extension |
| 2 | More marked increase in tone, but limb is easily flexed |
| 3 | Considerable increases in tone, passive movement difficult |
| 4 | Limb rigid in flexion or extension |

Ashworth, B. (1964). Preliminary trial of carisoprodol in multiple sclerosis. *Practitioner*, 192, 540-542.

## APPENDIX 2

### Modified Ashworth Scale

| Grade | Description |
|-------|-------------|
| 0 | No increase in muscle tone |
| 1 | Slight increase in muscle tone, manifested by a catch and release or by minimal resistance at the end of the range of motion when the affected part(s) is(are) moved in flexion or extension |
| 1+ | Slight increase in muscle tone, manifested by a catch followed by minimal resistance through the remainder of the range of motion but the affected part(s) is(are) easily moved. |
| 2 | More marked increase in muscle tone through most of the range of movement, but the affected part(s) is easily moved. |
| 3 | Considerable increases in muscle tone, passive movement difficult |
| 4 | Affected part(s) is (are) rigid in flexion or extension |

Bohannon, R.W. & Smith, MB. (1987). Interrater reliability of a Modified Ashworth Scale of muscle spasticity. *Phys Ther*, 67, 206-207.

# APPENDIX 3

## *Tardieu Scale*

### Velocity of stretch

Vi: As slow as possible (minimizing stretch reflex).
V2: Speed of the limb segment falling under gravity.
V3: As fast as possible (faster than the rate of the natural drop of the limb segment under gravity).

### Quality of the muscle reaction (X)

0: No resistance through the course of the passive movement.
1: Slight resistance throughout the course of the passive movement with no clear catch at a precise angle.
2: Clear catch at a precise angle, interrupting the passive movement, followed by release.
3: Fatigable clonus (<10 s when maintaining pressure) occurring at a precise angle.
4: Unfatigable clonus ( >10 s when maintaining pressure) occurring at a precise angle

Tardieu, G. & Shentoub, S. & Delarue, R.A. (1954). La recherche d'une technique de measure de la spasticite. *Rev Neurol (Paris)*, 91, 143–144.

# APPENDIX 4

## *Multiple Sclerosis Spasticity Scale (MSSS-88)*

- This questionnaire asks how *bothered* you have been by your spasticity *in the past two weeks.*
- By spasticity, we mean muscle stiffness and spasms.
- By *bothered,* we mean how distressed or upset you have been by any of the following problems.
- For each statement, please circle the one number that best describes how you feel.
- Please answer all questions, even if some seem rather similar to others or irrelevant to you.

## Section 1:

This section concerns muscle stiffness.

| As a result of your *spasticity,* how much in the past two weeks have you been bothered by: | Not at all bothered | A little bothered | Moderately bothered | Extremely bothered |
|---|---|---|---|---|
| 01. Stiffness when walking? | 1 | 2 | 3 | 4 |
| 02. Stiffness anywhere in your lower limbs? | 1 | 2 | 3 | 4 |
| 03. Stiffness when you are in the same position for a long time? | 1 | 2 | 3 | 4 |
| 04. Stiffness first thing in the morning? | 1 | 2 | 3 | 4 |
| 05. Tightness anywhere in your lower limbs? | 1 | 2 | 3 | 4 |
| 06. Your lower limbs feeling rigid? | 1 | 2 | 3 | 4 |
| 07. Stiffness when standing up? | 1 | 2 | 3 | 4 |
| 08. Tightness in your muscles? | 1 | 2 | 3 | 4 |
| 09. Stiffness that is unpredictable? | 1 | 2 | 3 | 4 |
| 10. Feeling that your muscles are pulling? | 1 | 2 | 3 | 4 |
| 11. Stiffness in your whole body? | 1 | 2 | 3 | 4 |
| 12. Your whole body feeling rigid? | 1 | 2 | 3 | 4 |

## Section :2

This section concerns pain and discomfort.

| As a result of your *spasticity*, how much in the past two weeks have you been bothered by: | Not at all bothered | A little bothered | Moderately bothered | Extremely bothered |
|---|---|---|---|---|
| 13. Feeling restricted and uncomfortable? | 1 | 2 | 3 | 4 |
| 14. Feeling uncomfort sitting for along time ? | 1 | 2 | 3 | 4 |
| 15. Painful or uncomfortable spasms? | 1 | 2 | 3 | 4 |
| 16. Pain when in the same position for too long? | 1 | 2 | 3 | 4 |
| 17. Feeling uncomfortable lying down for a long time? | 1 | 2 | 3 | 4 |
| 18. Difficulties finding a comfortable position to sleep in bed? | 1 | 2 | 3 | 4 |
| 19. Pain in the muscles on getting out of bed in the morning? | 1 | 2 | 3 | 4 |
| 20. Pain in the muscles provoked by movement? | 1 | 2 | 3 | 4 |
| 21. Constant pain in the muscles? | 1 | 2 | 3 | 4 |

## Section 3:

This section concerns muscle spasms.

| As a result of your *spasticity*, how much in the past two weeks have you been bothered by: | Not at all bothered | A little bothered | Moderately bothered | Extremely bothered |
|---|---|---|---|---|
| 22. Spasms that come on unpredictably? | 1 | 2 | 3 | 4 |
| 23. Powerful or strong spasms? | 1 | 2 | 3 | 4 |
| 24. Spasms when first getting out of bed in the morning? | 1 | 2 | 3 | 4 |
| 25. Spasms provoked by changing positions? | 1 | 2 | 3 | 4 |
| 26. Spasms provoked by movement? | 1 | 2 | 3 | 4 |
| 27. Spasms where your leg kicks out in front of you? | 1 | 2 | 3 | 4 |
| 28. Spasms provoked by certain positions? | 1 | 2 | 3 | 4 |
| 29. Spasms disturbing sleep? | 1 | 2 | 3 | 4 |
| 30. Spasms when doing certain tasks? | 1 | 2 | 3 | 4 |
| 31. Spasms when traveling over bumps or cobbles? | 1 | 2 | 3 | 4 |
| 32. Spasms where your knees pull up? | 1 | 2 | 3 | 4 |

| | | | | |
|---|---|---|---|---|
| 33. Spasms causing legs to hit things? | 1 | 2 | 3 | 4 |
| 34. Spasms provoked by touch? | 1 | 2 | 3 | 4 |
| 35. Spasms pushing you out of a chair or wheelchair? | 1 | 2 | 3 | 4 |

## Section 4:

This section concerns the effect of spasticity on your daily activities.

As a result of your *spasticity,* how much have you been limited in your ability over the past two weeks to carry out the following daily activities? (please circle 4 if you are unable to do the activity).

| | Not at all limited | A little limited | Moderately limited | Extremely limited |
|---|---|---|---|---|
| 36. Putting on your socks or shoes ? | 1 | 2 | 3 | 4 |
| 37. Doing housework such as cooking or cleaning? | 1 | 2 | 3 | 4 |
| 38. Getting in and out of a car? | 1 | 2 | 3 | 4 |
| 39. Getting in and out of shower and/or bath? | 1 | 2 | 3 | 4 |
| 40. Sitting up in bed? | 1 | 2 | 3 | 4 |
| 41. Getting into or out of bed? | 1 | 2 | 3 | 4 |
| 42. Turning over in bed? | 1 | 2 | 3 | 4 |

**(Continued)**

| | | | | |
|---|---|---|---|---|
| 43. Getting into or out of a chair? | 1 | 2 | 3 | 4 |
| 44. Getting dressed or undressed? | 1 | 2 | 3 | 4 |
| 45. Getting on or off the toilet seat? | 1 | 2 | 3 | 4 |
| 46. Drying yourself with a towel? | 1 | 2 | 3 | 4 |

## Section 5:

This section concerns the effect of spasticity on your ability to walk.

If you <u>cannot take any steps</u> at all, even with help, please tick this box and ignore questions 47 to 56.

| As a result of your _spasticity_, how much in the past two weeks have you been bothered by: | Not at all bothered | A little bothered | Moderately bothered | Extremely bothered |
|---|---|---|---|---|
| 47. Difficulties walking smoothly? | 1 | 2 | 3 | 4 |
| 48. Being slow when walking? | 1 | 2 | 3 | 4 |
| 49. Having to concentrate on your walking? | 1 | 2 | 3 | 4 |
| 50. Having to increase the effort needed for you to walk? | 1 | 2 | 3 | 4 |
| 51. Being slow when going up or down stairs? | 1 | 2 | 3 | 4 |
| 52. Being clumsy when walking? | 1 | 2 | 3 | 4 |
| 53. Tripping over or stumbling when walking? | 1 | 2 | 3 | 4 |

| | | | | |
|---|---|---|---|---|
| 54. Feeling like you are walking through treacle? | 1 | 2 | 3 | 4 |
| 55. Losing your confidence to walk? | 1 | 2 | 3 | 4 |
| 56. Feeling embarrassed to walk? | 1 | 2 | 3 | 4 |

## *Section 6:*

This section concerns the effect of spasticity on your body movements.

| As a result of your *spasticity*, how much in the past two weeks have you been bothered by: | Not at all bothered | A little bothered | Moderatel y bothered | Extremely bothered |
|---|---|---|---|---|
| 57. Difficulties moving freely? | 1 | 2 | 3 | 4 |
| 58. Difficulties moving smoothly? | 1 | 2 | 3 | 4 |
| 59. Limited range of movement? | 1 | 2 | 3 | 4 |
| 60. Difficulties moving parts of your body? | 1 | 2 | 3 | 4 |
| 61. Difficulties bending your limbs? | 1 | 2 | 3 | 4 |
| 62. Your body being resistant to movement? | 1 | 2 | 3 | 4 |
| 63. Your body or limbs feeling locked? | 1 | 2 | 3 | 4 |

**(Continued)**

| | | | | |
|---|---|---|---|---|
| 64. Awkward or jerky movement? | 1 | 2 | 3 | 4 |
| 65. Difficulties straightening your limbs? | 1 | 2 | 3 | 4 |
| 66. Difficulties relaxing parts of your body? | 1 | 2 | 3 | 4 |
| 67. No control over your body? | 1 | 2 | 3 | 4 |

## *Section 7:*

This section concerns the effect of spasticity on your feelings.

| As a result of your <u>spasticity</u>, how much in the past two weeks have you been bothered by: | Not at all bothered | A little bothered | Moderately bothered | Extremely bothered |
|---|---|---|---|---|
| 68. Feeling frustrated? | 1 | 2 | 3 | 4 |
| 69. Feeling less confident in yourself? | 1 | 2 | 3 | 4 |
| 70. Feeling inadequate? | 1 | 2 | 3 | 4 |
| 71. Feeling low? | 1 | 2 | 3 | 4 |
| 72. Feeling irritated? | 1 | 2 | 3 | 4 |

| 73. Feeling angry? | 1 | 2 | 3 | 4 |
|---|---|---|---|---|
| 74. Feeling depressed? | 1 | 2 | 3 | 4 |
| 75. Loss of self-worth? | 1 | 2 | 3 | 4 |
| 76. Feeling like a failure? | 1 | 2 | 3 | 4 |
| 77. Feeling frightened? | 1 | 2 | 3 | 4 |
| 78. Crying (tearful)? | 1 | 2 | 3 | 4 |
| 79. Feeling panicky? | 1 | 2 | 3 | 4 |
| 80. Feeling nervous? | 1 | 2 | 3 | 4 |

## Section 8:

This section concerns the effect of spasticity on your social functioning

| As a result of your _spasticity_, how much in the past two weeks have you been bothered by: | Not at all bothered | A little bothered | Moderately bothered | Extremely bothered |
|---|---|---|---|---|
| 81. Difficulties going out? | 1 | 2 | 3 | 4 |
| 82. Feeling isolated? | 1 | 2 | 3 | 4 |
| 83. Feeling vulnerable? | 1 | 2 | 3 | 4 |

**(Continued)**

| | | | | |
|---|---|---|---|---|
| 84. Difficulties finding energy for other people? | 1 | 2 | 3 | 4 |
| 85. Feeling reluctant to go out? | 1 | 2 | 3 | 4 |
| 86. Feeling less sociable? | 1 | 2 | 3 | 4 |
| 87. Difficulties with relationships with other family members? | 1 | 2 | 3 | 4 |
| 88. Difficulties interacting with people? | 1 | 2 | 3 | 4 |

Hobart, J.C & Riazi A. & Thompson, A.J.& Styles, I.M. & Ingram, W. & Vickery P.J. & Warner M. & Fox P.J. & Zajicek J.P. (2006). Getting the measure of spasticity in Multiple Sclerosis: the Multiple Sclerosis Spasticity Scale (MSSS-88). *Brain,* 129, 224-34.

# APPENDIX 5

## *Numeric Rating Scale*

On a scale of 0 to 10, please indicate your level of your level of spasticity over the last 24 Hours

Please tick ( ) 1 box only

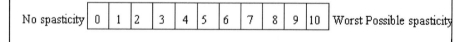

No spasticity | 0 | 1 | 2 | 3 | 4 | 5 | 6 | 7 | 8 | 9 | 10 | Worst Possible spasticity

Farrar, J.T. & Troxel, A.B. & Stott, C. & Duncombe, P. & Jensen, M.P. (2008) Validity, Reliability, and Clinical Importance of Change in a 0–10 Numeric Rating Scale measure of spasticity: a post hoc analysis of a randomized, double-blind, placebo-controlled trial. *Clinical Therapeutics,* 30(5), 224-234.

## APPENDIX 6

*Spasm Frequency Scale*

| Score | Description |
|-------|-------------|
| 0. | None. |
| 1. | No spontaneous spasms; but vigorous sensory or motor stimulation results in spasm. |
| 2. | Occasional spontaneous spasms or easily induced spasms. |
| 3. | Greater than one but less than ten spontaneous spasms per hour. |
| 4. | Greater than ten spontaneous spasms per hour. |

Pedersen, E. & Klemar B. & Torring J. (1979). Counting of Flexor Spasm. *Acta Neural Scand*, 60, 164-169.

## APPENDIX 7

*Penn Spasm Frequency Scale*

| Score | Description |
|-------|-------------|
| 0. | No Spasms. |
| 1. | Spasms Induced By Only Stimulation. |
| 2. | Spasms Occurring Less Than Once Per Hour. |
| 3. | Spasms Occurring More Than Once Per Hour. |
| 4. | Spasm Occurring More Than Ten Times Per Hour. |

Penn, R.D. & Savoy S.D. & Corcos D. & Latash M. & Gottlieb G. & Parke B. & et al. (1989). Intrathecal baclofen for severe spasticity. *N Engl J Med*, 320, 1517-1521.

## APPENDIX 8

*Hacettepe University Department of Physical Therapy, Neurological Rehabilitation Unit : Spastic Patient Assessment Form*

Name-Surname :_____

Gender: _____

Age: _____

Duration of disease : _____

MS type: _____

EDSS: _____

MAS Score  (0 to 4)

|  | Visit I Left | Visit I Right | Visit II Left | Visit II Right |
|---|---|---|---|---|
| Upper Extremity Proksimal |  |  |  |  |
| Upper Extremity Distal |  |  |  |  |
| Lower Extremity Proksimal |  |  |  |  |
| Lower Extremity Distal |  |  |  |  |

## *Numeric Rating Scale*

●━━━━━━━━━━━━━━━━━━━━━━━━━━━━━━━━━━━━●

0                                                                          10

On a scale of 0 to 10, please indicate your level of your level of spasticity over the last 24 Hours.

## *Goniometric Measurement*

|  | Visit I Left | Visit I Right | Visit II Left | Visit II Right |
|---|---|---|---|---|
| Upper Extremity Proksimal |  |  |  |  |
| Upper Extremity Distal |  |  |  |  |
| Lower Extremity Proksimal |  |  |  |  |
| Lower Extremity Distal |  |  |  |  |

* Please write active and passive limitations of joints caused by spasticity.

*Posture Analyses*

|  | Visit I | Visit II |
|---|---|---|
| Anterior |  |  |
| Posterior |  |  |
| Lateral |  |  |

*Observational Gait Analyses*

|  | Visit I | Visit II |
|---|---|---|
| Steppage gait |  |  |
| Scissor gait |  |  |
| Circumduction gait |  |  |

*Please put on (+) that is your patients gait pattern.

*Pathological Reflex Assessment*

|  | Visit I | Visit II |
|---|---|---|
| Babinski |  |  |
| Clonus |  |  |
| Hoffmann |  |  |
| Tramner |  |  |
| Palmomental |  |  |

*Please put on (+) if the pathological reflexes exist and put on (-) if it does not exist

*Muscle Strength Test*

|  | Visit I | Visit II |
|---|---|---|
| • M. ilopusuas |  |  |
| • M. guluteus maximus |  |  |
| • M. guluteus medius |  |  |
| • M. internal rotators |  |  |
| • M. quadriceps femoris |  |  |
| • M. hamstrings |  |  |
| • M. gastrosoleus |  |  |
| • M. tibialis anterior |  |  |
| • M. peroneals |  |  |

## (Continued)

| | | |
|---|---|---|
| • M. tibialis posterior | | |
| • M. extansor hallucis longus | | |
| • Lateral abdominals | | |

### *Total Point of Questionares*

| | Visit I | Visit II |
|---|---|---|
| MSSS 88 | | |
| Penn spasm Frequency Score | | |
| Berg Balance Score | | |
| FIM Score | | |
| SF 36 | | |

### *Superficial Sensory Assessment*

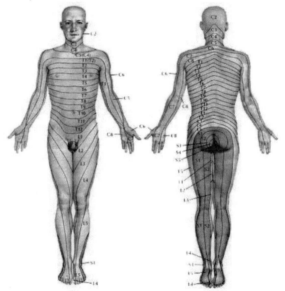

Please put on X if patient has sensory problem.

Others: _____

Physiotherapist name : _____

Signature: _____

*Chapter 8*

# PHYSIOTHERAPY APPLICATIONS

## *Kadriye Armutlu and Ayla Fil*

Hacettepe University, Faculty of Health Sciences, Department of Physical
Therapy and Rehabilitation, Neurological Rehabilitation Unit
06100/Ankara/TURKEY

## 8.1. ABSTRACT

There are a number of physiotherapy methods in clinical practice for the
management of spasticity based on neurophysiological and
neurodevelopmental principles. In general, these applications are divided into
two groups.

Direct approaches, such as cold application, passive exercises, stretching
exercises, neural mobilization, positioning, manual therapeutic approaches,
vibration, electrical stimulation, biofeedback and kinesiotape applications,
aim at spastic muscle or the antagonist muscle and focus on the inhibition of
spastic muscle.

Indirect approaches that affect spasticity by aiming at posture and
components of the movements and body segments focus on the facilitation of
antagonist muscle. Indirect approaches are neurodevelopmental treatment
methods, proprioceptive neuromuscular facilitation, body image and sensory
integration training, stimulation of vestibular system, hippotherapy,
hydrotherapy and reflexiology.

Physical therapists should evaluate patients correctly and determine their
necessity. Different types of approaches can be used together to manage
spasticity. Treatment prescription should be planned according to patient's
necessity.

Key words: spasticity, physical therapy, exercise, neuro-developmental treatments, sensory-motor integration, manual therapy, electrical stimulation, vestibular stimulation.

## 8.2 INTRODUCTON

MS differs from the diseases like stroke, SCI, CP, etc. in terms of symptom diversity and complexity, clinical signs and its progressive character. Spasticity is managed within a stabile disease profile in patients suffering from these diseases, whereas an MS patient with spasticity has unpredictable relapses and the disease continues to progress, requiring a flexible physical therapy programme and treatment goals. The physiotherapist—as the heart of the rehabilitation team—has to encounter other symptoms and problems of MS along with spasticity. In general, the objective of the therapist during this encounter should be as follows:

### 8.2.1. Beginning and Early Phase (1 to 5.5 EDSS)

Patients who are able to walk short distances unsupervised:

- Inhibition of spasticity.
- Development of postural control.
- Enhancing muscle strength.
- Facilitation of normal movement components and patterns.
- Development of normal posture balance, walk and coordination.
- Instruction of the patient about the disease and principles that he should be aware of during daily life (avoiding heat and infections, etc.).
- Development of home-exercise habit.

*Objective: Improvement of patient's functional level.*

### 8.2.2. Middle phase (6 to 7 EDSS)

Patients who are able to walk short distances by unilateral or bilateral support:

- Management of spasticity and reducing its effects.

- Maintenance of muscle strength and enhancing it as far as possible.
- Maintenance of ROM.
- Maintaining the functionality of proximal muscle groups.
- Maintenance of lung capacity by use of chest physiotherapy applications
- Instructing the patient about the energy conservation in ADLs (activities of daily life) and compensation techniques. Also choosing proper self-support devices in order to reduce energy consumption to a minimum degree.
- Home adjustments.
- Maintenance of patient's mobility as far as possible by choosing proper walk supports and orthosis.

*Objective: Maintenance of patient's functional level and postponing the wheelchair use as long as possible.*

## 8.2.3. Advanced Phase (7.5 to 9.5 EDSS)

Patients who are confined to wheelchair and bed:

- Trying to prevent the contractures and deformities resulting from spasticity.
- Instructing the patient about the proper wheelchair design and wheelchair exercises.
- Choosing the proper bed.
- Avoiding bed complications (lung infections, decubitus ulcers, etc.).
- Instruction of proper transfer methods.
- Home adjustments.

*Objective: Avoidance of complications resulting from spasticity and immobility; prolonging the survival period.*

Specifically, the management/inhibition of spasticity is used for reducing energy consumption, maintaining posture, keeping hygiene, sustaining walk and mobility, decreasing the frequency of pain and spasms and consequently improving the functional capacity. What is to be emphasized in this point of view is not only the inhibition of spastic muscle but also the strengthening of antagonist muscle by using the proper techniques during this relative inhibition.

**ATTENTION!**
If the strengthening process of the affected muscle is neglected, there will be no significant improvement in functional recovery.

There are a number of physiotherapy methods in clinical practice for the management of spasticity based on neurophysiological and neurodevelopmental principles. In general, these applications are divided into two groups: direct approaches that focus on the inhibition of spastic muscle and indirect approaches that affect spasticity by paying attention to posture and components of the movements with body segments, focusing on the facilitation of antagonist muscle. Some techniques involve local applications and some involve extensive applications affecting wider body segments. However, when spasticity is moderated by use of local applications, a general relaxation may occur in the whole body (Table 1).

**Table 1. Physiotherapy Approaches**

| Direct/Local Approaches | Indirect/general Approaches |
| --- | --- |
| Cold application | Neurodevelopmental treatment |
| Passive exercises | methods (Bobath, Johnstone, Rood |
| Stretching exercises | approaches) |
| Neural mobilization | Proprioceptive neuromuscular |
| Orthotic Devices | facilitation (PNF) |
| Positioning | Body image and sensory integration |
| Manual therapeutic approaches (joint | training |
| and soft tissue mobilization-deep | Stimulation of vestibular system |
| massage) | Hippotherapy |
| Vibration | Hydrotherapy |
| Electrical Stimulation | Reflexology |
| Biofeedback | |
| Kinesiotape applications | |

## 8.3. DIRECT/LOCAL APPROACHES

Direct/local physiotherapy applications have numerous objectives that include the inhibition of spastic muscles, restoration of shortened structures, strengthening of weak muscles and development of normal postural tone. The therapist should keep in mind that the inhibition of the spastic muscle for short duration depends relatively on the frequency and severity of the spasticity and the muscle stiffness. Even a partial inhibition is sufficient for the antagonist movement. During this limited period of time, the physiotherapist should stimulate the antagonist muscle by using proper facilitation methods as much as possible. This stimulation leads to the contraction of antagonist muscle resulting in a reciprocal inhibition and allowing further inhibition of spastic agonist muscle with the effect of neural factors.

It is known that there are numerous direct approaches in physical therapy practice. Determination of the proper method depends on the patient profile and the clinical environment itself.

## 8.3.1. Cold Application

### Prolonged Cold Application

The prolonged cold application aims at reducing pain and hypertonus. Long-term cold application decreases the amplitude of motor action potentials, nerve transmission speed, impulses that originate from sensory afferents and the activity of muscle fibers. In addition, metabolic velocity of spastic muscle exposed to cold decreases. These factors altogether may cause the inhibition of monosynaptic stretch reflex. Moreover, due to its effect on pain reduction, cold application inhibits flexor spasms triggered by pain.

The cold application method is common in clinical practice by physiotherapists due to its above-mentioned effects on decreasing the intensity of spasticity. When various studies on cold application in literature are reviewed, the applications performed in different levels, periods and forms stand out.

Cold application may be applied by use of ice packs, cold air, cold spray, ice massage and cold baths. However, application of cold by use of cold air or spray may increase the intensity of spasticity [1].

In an experiment on rabbits conducted by Lee et al., cold air was applied for 30 and 60 minutes to decrease the inner muscle temperature to 32.5, 30 and 25 degrees. As a result, between 30- and 60-minute periods, applications causing the temperature decrease to 30 degrees proved to be more efficient. But when the temperature was decreased to 25 degrees, a total nerve block occurred [2]. According to Prince and Lehmann, cold application should be performed until inner muscle temperature is decreased [3]. Bell and Lehmann conveyed that inner muscle temperature decreased to 31 degrees after 20 minutes of ice pack application [4].

Studies prove that intensity of spasticity does not abate unless there is a decrease in body temperature; therefore, applications lasting for 20 to 30 minutes, decreasing inner muscle temperature to 30 degrees and slowing down the nerve transmission, are preferred. According to Lehmann and deLauter, duration of the application may vary depending on the subcutaneous fatty tissue [5].

It is known that changes in temperature directly affect MS symptoms. An increase in temperature usually has negative outcomes on functions, whereas positive developments occur when temperature is decreased. It is assumed that low temperature/cold often reduces fatigue and spasticity and increases muscle strength and mobility [6].

In research by Petrili et al., 191 MS patients were questioned about the effects of temperature on their clinical symptoms like spasticity, fatigue, difficulties in walking, etc. Findings were as follows: 147 patients conveyed that they were negatively affected, 104 patients' conditions worsened with high temperature and 82 patients felt relaxation in the low temperature. On the other hand, 20 patients stated that low temperature resulted in symptom regression, and 19 of these patients conveyed that they felt better in high temperature [7].

In a study made by Chiara et al. on 14 MS patients, the effects of cold bath (24°C) on the severity of spasticity and on oxygen consumption was studied. Patients were seated in a 35.5cm² hydrotherapy tank for 20 minutes. As a result, patients' spasticity was aggravated on MAS scores. However, this increase was not considered statistically significant. Furthermore, following the application, it was observed that most of the patients trembled although their body temperatures were normal [6].

Another study was conducted by Nilsagard et al. on 43 MS patients who were sensitive to heat. The patients were clothed in cold clothes, and their 10- and 30-meter timed walk, oral temperature, spasticity, standing balance, timed "up and go" test, and nine-hole peg test performances were measured. Although there was no objective alteration observed on spasticity; subjects stated that they were affected by the application positively. Oral temperature measurements showed no signs of alteration during the experiment [8].

Consequently, 20- to 30-minute application of cold packs (easily obtained and applied) on spastic muscle generally proves to be a reliable method to decrease the severity of spasticity on MS patients. However, the cold application may not be the proper method to use on patients with sense deprivation, autonomic dysfunction (feeling cold, hypothermia and reflex sympathetic dystrophia), irritation to cold application, and frequent urinary tract infections.

**ATTENTION!**
Cold application may not be an appropriate method for some patients.

### Short-Term Cold Application

The short-term cold application is used to stimulate the antagonist of the spastic muscle. Sponge-covered ice cubes are compressed rapidly for three to five seconds on the dermatome of target muscle. The objective is to stimulate the related receptors and inhibit the spastic antagonist muscle through reciprocal inhibition. However, the short-term cold application may not lead to desired outcomes in some cases. Cold is regarded as a potential threat by the nervous system. Sudden exposure of cold may activate contraction in the muscle in order to avoid this "threat." If the patient has pervasive lower extremity extensor spasticity with no complaints of flexor spasms, stimulation of traction reflex may be advantageous [9]. On the other hand, if the patient has spasticity affecting flexor muscles and complaints of flexor spasms, the short-term cold application may cause an aggravation of these symptoms.

## 8.3.2. Passive Exercises

Passive exercises are applied to patients with spasticity and on patients who are unable to perform active movements due to impaired muscles in order to maintain muscle length, improve ROM, and increase proprioceptive senses with the sense of movement [10]. Passive exercises are usually applied on patients with medium or high EDSS scores (EDSS 5.5>), whose ability of mobilization is quite limited. Passive exercises may become risky when this partial immobility and osteoporothic effects of steroids on bones are considered. Possible side-effects are linear fractures in the head and neck of the femur and avascular necrosis of the femoral head.

**ATTENTION!**
In cases of osteoporothic patients, the physical therapist should apply passive exercise within pain limits, avoid forcing the hip in hyperadduction and internal rotation.

The patient, his relatives and caretakers should be instructed about avoiding the risks during the application of home exercises. As long as it is applied carefully considering the mentioned risks, passive exercises are a good option for moderating the effects of spasticity on muscles and joints.

The primal effect of passive exercise on spastic muscle occurs by way of thixotropy. The term thixotrophy has been applied to substances that can be changed from gel to solution after being stirred. The muscle acts as a thixotrophic substance in that its stiffness depends on the history of limb movement [11]. Active or passive movement reduces the sarcoplasmic viscosity of the spastic muscle, thus leading to lesser resistance to passive movement. Passive exercise may be combined with the other antispastic applications as a supplementary method. In order to not to aggravate spasticity, speed and duration of the exercise and the manipulation of body parts should be observed carefully.

In literature, there is only one study regarding the effects of passive exercises on MS patients—ten MS patients and ten healthy persons participated in this study, which was conducted by Nuyens et al. The purpose of this study was to investigate the effect of movement repetitions on resistive torque during passive isokinetic dynamometry of the knee and to determine the role of electromyographic activity in the stretched muscles on the torque measurements. During series of ten flexion and extension movements of the knee at 60, 180 and 300 degrees/s, torque and electromyographic activity in the stretched muscles were registered. The patients with hypertonia presented a significantly larger torque reduction ($p < 0.05$) than the control subjects in all test conditions except for repeated knee flexion at 300 degrees/s [12].

According to the findings of a study conducted by Nuyens et al., passive repetitive isokinetic movements decreased muscle tonicity in stroke patients [13].

### 8.3.3. Stretching

Stretching is used frequently to maintain soft tissue flexibility and to prevent contractures. Tension is applied on soft tissues during stretching. Muscles, tendons, connective tissues, skin, vessels and nerves are the structures under tension. Different stretching forms and stretch tensions may be applied on different structures. Stretching may alter the viscoelastibility and excitability of the muscle [14]. Alterations in muscle excitability depend on the responses of proprioceptors to different stretch types.

Stretching can be applied both manually and mechanically. In general literature, stretching is classified in four groups: static, dynamic, ballistic and passive.

***Slow And Prolonged Stretching***

This type of stretching is used for two purposes: restoration of normal length of the shortened muscle and inhibition of spastic muscle with facilitation of antagonist muscle via autogenetic inhibition by keeping the tendon under tension while stretching the spastic muscle.

Stretching by using manual or isokinetic devices can be applied for a short period of time (five minutes approximately).

Manuel stretching is applied by the physical therapist during the supervised treatment; however, patients with minimal impairment should be instructed for self-stretching. In addition to self-stretching and supervised stretching, stretch of specific muscles **several times a day should be applied by patient's relatives** and caretakers. Below are the rules to be followed during stretching:

- If there are no contraindications, cold should be applied to spastic muscles. This increases the stimulation threshold of the spindle and inhibits the pain sense partially.
- In order not to stimulate the velocity-related responses of spasticity, stretching should be applied very slowly, recessed at the point of resistance and held until the resistance is declined; then move on to the pain limit and hold there for a few minutes.

- If patient's active participation is high and his antagonist muscles are not too weak, stretching should be initialized by the patient and supervised from the point of resistance.
- If stretching of more than one muscle is required, it should be applied within a pattern. To avoid distress, more tension should be applied to proximal structures, and distals should be let loose slightly. When the patient adapts to the stretch and his distress is decreased, distal structures should be exposed to the same degree of tension as proximals (i.e., if the therapist plans the stretching of hamstrings, gastrocnemius and long finger flexors, he should apply the stretch first on hamstrings, then on gastrocnemius and finally on finger flexors)
- Stretching is applied to attain inhibition; therefore, it should never be applied ballistically (figures 1 and 2).
- During self-stretching, the patient should follow the same rules and perform the movements in different positions such as standing, sitting or lying.

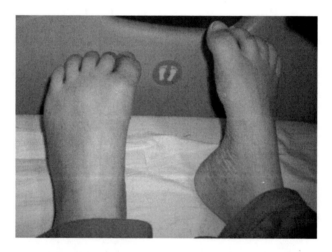

Figure 1. Bilateral spastic foot.

The shortness of duration results in a temporary inhibition, which is insufficient in altering the soft tissue to a desired length. For patients with severe spasticities, stretching by using orthosis or positioning is regarded to be more practical considering the high resistance of muscles. In such cases, the physical therapist may have difficulties when encountering the resistance and may have occupational injuries.

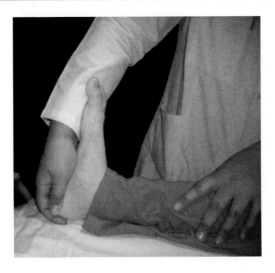

Figure 2. Manual Passive Stretch.

In textbooks, stretching stands out as the foremost-advised technique for MS symptom management, however, when literature is surveyed, there are quite few studies concerning stretching exercises. Such a study was conducted by Brar et al., on MS patients, lasting for four weeks. The study showed that stretching applied on each muscle group everyday for 1.5 minutes was deficient in decreasing spasticity [15].

Another study was conducted by Giovanelli et al. on 38 MS patients who were under botulinum toxin treatment for the moderation of spasticity. Patients were divided into two groups. Active and passive strengthening and stretching exercises were applied to the treatment group, whereas the control group did not receive any physical therapy treatments. At the end of the 12-week programme, a significant decrease in MAS scores of treatment group—compared with the control group—was observed [16].

Other studies were frequently conducted on stroke patients. Such a study was carried out by Yeh et al. During this study, ankle plantar flexors were pushed from neutral position to five degrees of dorsiflexion for 30 minutes by using constant-torque prolonged muscle stretching technique. As a result, ROM was improved and both the elastic and viscoelastic components of the spastic muscle were affected by the stretch [17]. Another study by the same researcher compared the effects of constant-torque prolonged muscle stretching technique with constant-angle prolonged muscle stretching technique on spasticity. These techniques were applied randomly on ankle muscles of 30 stroke patients for a period of one week each. The outcome of both techniques was a decrease in elastic and viscotic components of the spastic muscles. Furthermore, it was stated that stretching against torque turned out to be more efficient than stretching against angle; therefore, application of constant-torque prolonged muscle stretching technique should be preferred instead of other conventional stretching methods [18].

Stretching exercises should be both rhythmic and repetitive and also accord with proprioceptive facilitation techniques aiming at developing motor control [19].


### *Quick Stretching*

It is used for the facilitation of antagonist of the spastic muscle. Stretch degree should be determined in accordance with the fiber types of the weakened antagonist muscle. The aim is to enhance the inhibition of spastic muscle through reciprocal inhibition and increase the response of weak antagonist muscle to strengthening exercises through stimulation.


## 8.3.4. Neural Mobilization

Neural mobilization is also known as Maitland and Butler technique. It is based on the viewpoint that "the peripheral and central nervous systems need to be considered as one since they form a continuous tissue tract" [20.21]. Neural mobilization is a treatment modality used in relation to both orthopedic and nervous system pathologies. In normal circumstances, neural tissue is relatively mobile within the neural capsule. This mobility enables the nerve to actualize its optimal functions. Any injury concerning the connective tissues averts the neural tissue from moving within the surrounding tissue and increases intrinsic pressure, which may result in functional disorder. Neural mobilization restores the relative movement between neural and surrounding tissue and decreases the intrinsic pressure. Application of the gliding technique is used for the reduction of nerve adherence, dispersion of noxious fluids, increased neural vascularity and improvement of axoplasmic flow [22].

Alterations/stiffness in the intrinsic structure of spastic muscle exert pressure on peripheral nerves passing through the muscle, resulting in adhesion in the intrinsic structure of the nerve. This pathological outcome may gradually lead to loss of strength in the spastic muscle. Therefore, while applying stretch, the proper position for the nerve, innerving the muscle should be chosen and the muscle should be mobilized by rhythmic gliding. Treatment method is determined according to the level of immobility, pain range and the site of irritability.

Movements involved by the techniques are categorized in four grades. The physical therapist decides on the proper movement considering the character of pathology (irritable versus non-irritable). The Maitland grades can be listed as:

- **Grade I** A small amplitude movement performed close to the beginning of range.
- **Grade II** A large amplitude movement carried into the range. It's a movement that takes place in any degree of the range that is pain or resistance free.
- **Grade III** A large amplitude movement that moves up to the limit of range or into resistance.
- **Grade IV** A small amplitude movement performed close to the end of range or slightly into resistance [23, 24]. Treatment may be direct or indirect. Direct intervention refers to procedures directed to rebalancing the neuromusculoskeletal system through strengthening and increasing ROM to improve motor control. Indirect treatment includes the use of movement patterns, especially posture-based patterns. Nervous system changes, static and dynamic postural patterns often emerge as compensatory reactions to the problem state. Application of indirect method is more appropriate for restoring posture defects resulting from spasticity-related tension or stiffness.

Improved Proprioceptive Neuromuscular Facilitation (PNF) techniques make frequent use of neural mobilizations as well. Neural mobilization combined with PNF techniques are applied in forms of functional patterns.

Each nerve has a different mobilization position. The therapist should have a perfect knowledge of these positions and apply different combinations of movements accordingly. Nerves that require neural mobilization are often the ulnar, median, femoral and sciatic nerves, which innervate spastic muscles.

Although neural mobilization is an ancient technique with frequent use in clinical practice, there is no study concerning the effects of this technique on MS patients and MS spasticity in general literature. However, relying on clinical experiences, it can be claimed that neural mobilization application should be included in the treatment programmes of MS spasticity management.

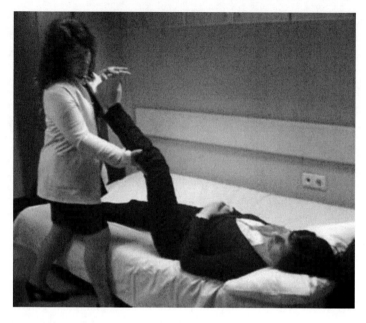

Figure 3. Neural mobilization of sciatic nerve.

## 8.3.5. Orthotic Devices

The effects of orthosis and splint usage on the inhibition of spasticity and on strengthening the weak muscles can be defined biomechanically or neurophysiologically. Orthotic devices are biomechanically effective on supporting body segments, improving function, limiting or enhancing movement and transferring body weight from one segment to another. Preventing or reducing the development of contractures by using orthosis/splint constitutes the most fundamental biomechanical effect. Furthermore, holding the lengthened spastic muscle in an antispastic position by using orthosis is assumed to result in facilitation of autogenetic inhibition and thus provide a decreased muscle tone.

Orthoses and splints can be categorized as static and dynamic. Static orthoses/splints are generally used to keep lower extremity in an antispastic position and to prevent contractures. Lower extremity static orthoses contribute to the walk function by holding the foot in a neutral position or in a degree of slight dorsiflexion.

*Lower Extremity Orthoses*

Foot and ankle orthoses (AFO) are the most commonly used orthotic devices for patients with lower extremity spasticities. AFOs have two subcategories:

## AFOs Made of Leather and Metal

These are specific types of shoes made of leather, with two metal bars in the sides supporting the leg, wrapped by a thigh band. Metal bars function as joints mounted on AFOs to allow the ankle move within the desired range or fix the ankle and avoid specific movement (figure 4). It has some advantages and disadvantages, such as:

- The foot feels comfortable in the shoe and sweating of the foot is avoided.
- Extra-modification apparatus are easily placed in the shoe.
- It is partially heavy.
- It is efficient only in a minimal spasticity.
- The metal bars have a non-cosmetic appearance.
- It controls only plantar flexion and dorsiflexion; therefore, deficient in other problems (pronation, etc.).

Relying on clinical experiences, it can be said that this type of AFO application is not suitable for MS patients. In cases of minimal spasticity, physical therapists tend to try alternative methods before deciding on the application orthosis, considering both advantages and the disadvantages (limitation of specific muscular movements) of orthosis usage. MS patient's dorsiflexors are able to move the feet upwards despite minimal gastronecmius spasticity. AFO application on such a patient is needless. Occasionally, extreme cases may arise that may require the use of AFO: despite minimal spasticity, severe dropped foot case may be observed resulting from disc hernia.

## Polypropylen AFO

These AFOs are highly preferred in the recent years (PAFO). PAFOs are custom-made by using a positive plaster model made in accordance with the measurements of the patient. Peak point of the orthosis may be produced with a slight angle upwards for patients who have heavy contraction of toe flexors while walking. PAFOs can be categorized in two subcategories within themselves, according to the support they provide:

- Non-rigid PAFOs: Non-rigid PAFOs are applied to patients with rarely minimal and generally moderate gastro-soleus spasticities. The purpose of PAFO is to maintain control of the ankle and subtalar joints and fix the foot in the plantigrade position or in a degree of slight dorsiflexion (five degrees maximum). Non-rijid PAFOs can be applied in two formations depending on the knee joint condition and strength of quadriceps femoris. Posterior leaf PAFOs are suitable for patients with quadriceps femoris strength above three. Dorsiflexion angle up to five degrees enables the control of hypertonus in quadriceps femoris and prevents uncontrolled hyperextansion of the knee. On this account, it is important that the quadriceps femoris muscle has the strength to resist the bending/torsion moment generated in the knee by this angle. Joints can be inserted on posterior leaf PAFO when required, since some patients are unable to use or tolerate jointless orthoses. In such cases, orthosis should be designed with plantar flexion stoppers enabling dorsiflexion (figures 5 and 6). If the quadriceps femoris muscle is weak, dorsiflexion angle should be minimum. In cases with impaired knee extensors, anterior shell PAFO may be preferred [25]. However, support point of anterior shell PAFOs is on the tibial surface, which is an area deficient in soft tissue; therefore, PAFO may cause skin irritations and distress in some patients.

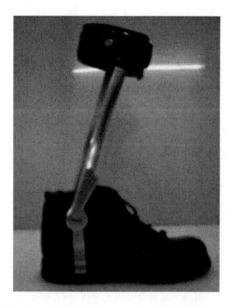

Figure 4. AFO made of leather and metal.

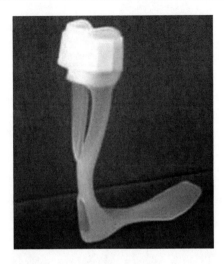

Figure 5. Posterior leaf PAFO.

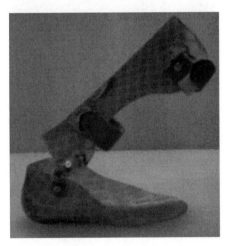

Figure 6. Jointless posterior leaf PAFO.

- Rigid PAFOs: In order to prevent plantar flexion and inversion of foot in patients with severe spasticity, rigid PAFO should be applied. If it is to be used during walking, PAFO should be placed behind the malleolars, and ventral part of the orthosis may be left uncovered. PAFOs with more coverage may be preferred for night use. When using this type of PAFO, pressure may be applied through the sides of Achilles tendon and under the metatarsal head. Pressure applied to these two areas aggravate the inhibition of spastic muscle by enhancing autogenetic inhibition mechanisms (figure 7).

Rigid PAFOs should establish full-contact to the area applied. Therefore, correct measurements should be taken from the patient, points of distress should be fixed and the patient should be checked frequently following the application. In order to avoid pressure ulcers, the interior of the PAFO should be covered with a soft material.

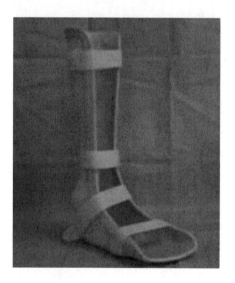

Figure 7. Rigid PAFO.

**ATTENTION!**
Rigid PAFO usage should be monitored with an extra care for the patients who have cutaneous sensory loss.

## Long Leg Orthosis (Knee ankle foot orthosis (KAFO))

It can be used for patients who do not have knee control to stand up and to help walking. It is made from rigid polypropylene material so that it can be light. It begins under the hip joint and extends to the ankle (Figure 8).

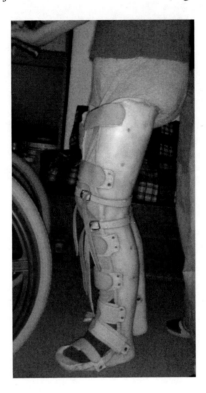

Figure 8. Long Leg Orthosis (KAFO).

## Upper Extremity Splints

Upper extremity splints are generally used to maintain hand and fingers in an antispastic position, generate inhibition and prevent contractions. Their use in functions is limited. Splints are usually applied to obtain abduction and semiflexion close to extension position in fingers; extension in wrists and neutral position in forearm [1].

There are two types of static wrist splints: dorsal and volar. Some physiotherapists prefer applying dorsal splints to patients with hyperactive grasp reflex in order not to contact volar surface. There is no definite scientific explanation regarding this kind of application. Duration of volar contact applied by splint would be long, which would lead to receptor adaptation and suppress hyperactive grasp reflex. Moreover, it is difficult to apply as well. Therefore, it may not be suitable for patients with severe spasticity. Volar splinter is easier to apply and to position (figure 9).

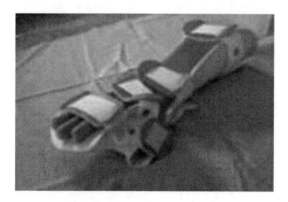

Figure 9. Static volar inhibitor hand splint.

Splint/orthosis application has its disadvantages and advantages. Unless the splint is applied properly, pressure wounds may occur in the area and the splint may become a painful stimulant itself and increase hypertonus. Orthotic devices increase perspiration; therefore, paying attention to hygiene is important. Sometimes, patients refuse to use splints for cosmetic reasons.

When general literature is reviewed, it is seen that there are no studies analyzing the effects of orthotic devices on MS patients with spasticity in particular. Existing studies usually focus on patients with stroke, cerebral palsy and spinal cord injuries. Their findings differ from one another. Some studies report that use of orthoses sustain walking and decrease spasticity [26, 27, 28] and some report that hand splints have no beneficial effects on spasticity [29].

## 8.3.6 Positioning

Positioning means to position the patient on chair or in bed. When done properly, meeting the needs of the patient, it enables ROM and stretching of the particular segments. Seating and bed positioning is important especially for patients with advanced MS (EDSS 7>).

During the process, weak muscles should be supported and spastic muscles be stretched. The tension obtained by positioning has long duration, which may lead to the stimulation of golgi tendon organ resulting in a decrease of muscle tonicity in the spastic muscle through autogenetic inhibition. Tension should be generated both in the tendon and the collagen structure of the muscle.

Stretching the segment that has a rigid contracture may cause distress and fatigue, which may lead to the aggravation of spasticity. If there is a presence of unrecoverable limitation, supporting rather than stretching should be preferred. Head and neck position may suppress tonic neck reflex and generate a decrease in muscle tonicity. Supine positions increase spasticity in extensors, lying prone increases spasticity in flexors; therefore, the patient should be examined carefully in order to determine the appropriate position.

According to the findings, supine lying is observed to increase the severity of spasticity, particularly in knee extensors [30].

Prone lying, on the other hand, usually causes an increase in flexor tonus, whereas lying on side has a neutral effect on muscle tonicity.

The areas affected from spasticity vary from one patient to another in MS; therefore, there is no definite configuration of positioning. It should be determined according to the tonicity observed and the needs of the patient. For instance, if a patient's spasticity is only in upper extremity, he doesn't have to be positioned rigidly in bed. However, if four extremities are stiffened, then all body segments should be positioned in the reverse direction of spasticity. Positioning and weight of the body segments can be used as a means of stretching the spastic muscles. When a patient with quadriceps femoris spasticity lays supine, knees bended and a roll is placed under the knees, the weight of the leg causes semiflexion in the knee and muscle tonicity decreases. To avoid hip and knee flexor contractions, 30 minutes prone lying two to three times a day, should be preferred with patients who have lower extremity flexor spasticity. Most patients who are not comfortable with this position should be persuaded by informing them about the importance of the application. During the positioning of spinal column and extremities, the head and neck should be maintained in the most neutral position.

Supplementary equipments like pillows and particular kinds of rolls may be used during positioning. For example, placing a t-shaped roll between the legs of a patient with adductor spasticity will be helpful in the positioning of the patient. In addition to that, the roll will keep adductor muscles stretched for a long duration, generating a moderation of spasticity (figures 10, 11).

## 8.3.7. Manual Therapy

Proprioceptive inputs deriving from the mechanoreceptors of joints, skin and fasia cause contractions in deep muscles (see chapter 6). Wyke categorized joint receptors in three types. Type 1 receptors are located in proximal joints and in apophysial joints in the cervical spine. Type 1 receptors adapt slowly to stress alterations occurring in the fibrous capsule they exist in, and their sensory threshold is low. Therefore, they are easily stimulated even when the joint is motionless. Effect of mechanoreceptors on muscle tonicity originates from the afferent discharges of type 1, type 2 and type 3 receptors. Type 1 and type 3 receptors are more important than those of type 2 [31].

Considering the information stated above, inhibition of spastic muscle, stabilization of extremity and facilitation of weak muscles can be achieved by use of manual techniques. Manual therapy targets muscles, tendons and joint receptors. Forms of manual application techniques are listed below:

### *Approximation*

Following the proper organization of body segments, pressure should applied throughout the segment axis. Pressure application should be carried on until a contraction in proximal muscles is felt or observed. Pressure and compression can be applied starting from the distal area to the proximal area of the body segment (properly positioned by the physiotherapist); or weight can be transferred from the proximal to the supported area (figures 13, 14, 15).

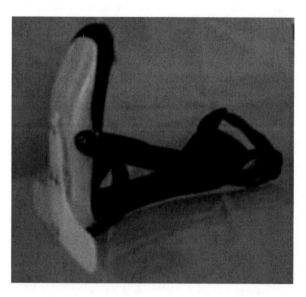

Figure 10. Equipment for position of foot.

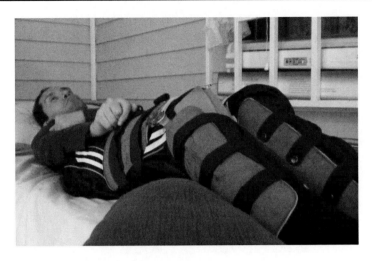

Figure 11. Bed positioning for flexor Spasticity.

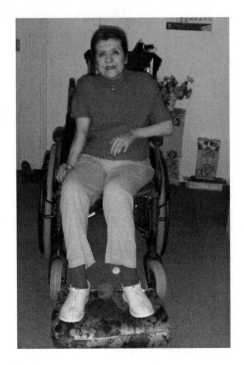

Figure 12. Seating positioning.

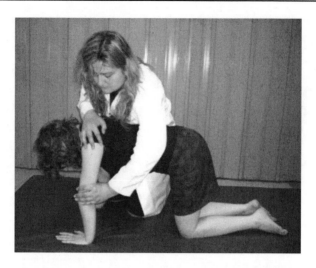

Figure 13. Approximation on the spastic.

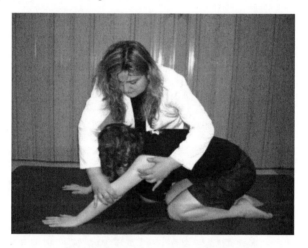

Figure 14. Approximat on with upper extremity weight-bearing activity.

In order to decrease spasticity in the lower extremity, weight can be transferred from the proximal pelvis to the leg fixed in an antispastic position. Additionally, transfer of weight from the knee to the foot when the patient is seated and approximation may help to decrease muscle tone in ankles. To moderate spasticity in the upper extremity, body weight should be transferred from the shoulder to the hand after positioning hands and elbows properly. This may decrease muscle tonicity in upper extremity and increase proximal muscle strength, resulting in the stimulation of normal movement and normal postural tonus. Weight can be transferred to the forearm instead of hands as well [32].

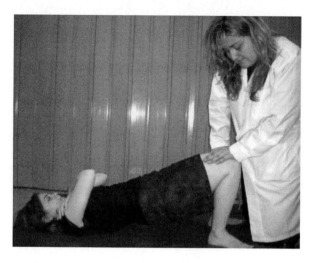

Figure 15. Approximation on the spastic lower extremity on the bridge position.

### Inhibitory Pressure

Pressure is used therapeutically to alter motor responses. Inhibitory pressure technique works when pressure is applied across the longitudinal axis of tendon. The therapist should continue applying pressure until the muscle is fully relaxed, without changing the point of pressure (figure 16).

Pressure is not merely effective on tendon but also on specific muscles when applied on specific bone margins. For instance, pressure applied on the medial calcaneus results in the inhibition of plantar flexors and facilitation of lateral dorsiflexors. Application of pressure on lateral calcaneus results in the inhibition plantar flexors and facilitation of medial dorsiflexors.

### Stretch Pressure and Stretch Release

Stretch pressure targets on muscle fiber. Pressure must be applied rapidly and sharply from the center of muscle trunk. In case of stimulation generated in the fiber, a slight inhibition of spastic muscle is achieved.

Stretch-release aims at the skin tissue. Sudden stretch applied to the skin covering antagonist of spastic muscle, stimulates cutaneous receptors that indirectly stimulate muscle fiber in return, resulting in the inhibition of spastic muscle.

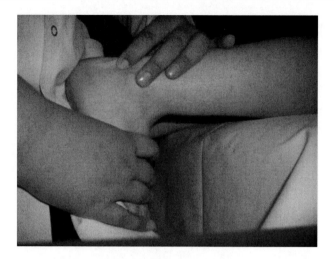

Figure 16. Inhibitor pressure on Achilles Tendon.

### Slow Stroking

Slow stroking over the paravertebral areas along the spine from the cervical through lumbar components will cause inhibition or decreased over activity of the sympathetic nervous system. Massage should be applied for three to five minutes at most, since prolonged stroking may cause rebounds in autonomic responses.

### Soft Tissue Mobilization

Soft tissue mobilization is composed of connective tissue manipulation and deep soft tissue massage. The goal of soft tissue mobilization application to spastic muscles where non-neural component is prominent, to the corresponding fasia and to the skin, is to attain the normal length and elasticity of the tissues (figure 17). In order to moderate the sense of pain, prolonged cold application may be employed prior to connective tissue manipulation. Deep massage and manipulation should be applied for approximately five minutes, until a relative softness in muscle tissue is obtained.

The application of massage to hand and foot sole may generate an increase in proprioceptive inputs and reduce the increase in reflexive tonus by way of desensitization. For instance, massage application to the foot sole of a patient who has positive support reaction in his foot (before he stands up), combined with application of mobilization to posterior crural muscle group and the Achilles tendon will desensitize muscles against intrinsic and extrinsic stimuli and moderate this unwanted reaction [25] (figures 18 and 19).

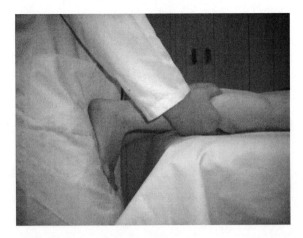

Figure 17. Deep friction massage for gastrosoleus muscle.

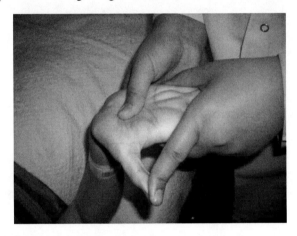

Figure 18. Deep friction massage for hand.

## *Joint Mobilisation*

Joint mobilization is applied to secure normal ROM in the joints that are limited by spasticity [33]. Techniques such as Cyriax's, McKenzie, etc. may also be used for this purpose. Starting the antispastic application with neck mobilization is important for the regulation of muscle tonicity. It is known that type 1 mechanoreceptors located in the neck are effective in managing muscle tonicity. Therefore, starting the treatment with neck mobilization will stimulate receptors in this area and enable the regulation of muscle tonicity. Furthermore, neck mobilization is believed to decrease the activation of sympathetic truncus, thereby contributing to the regulation of whole body muscle tone. Neck mobilization of MS patients should be maintained within the limits of grade 1, and reactions of the patient during the application should be observed closely (figures 20 and 21).

Studies considering the highly preferred manual therapy technique often used in musculo-skeletal problems cannot be found in MS literature.

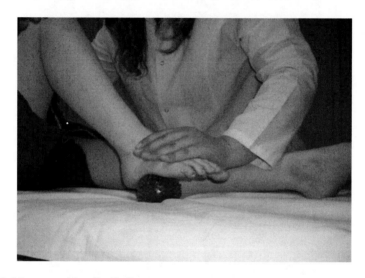

Figure 19. Massage with reflex ball.

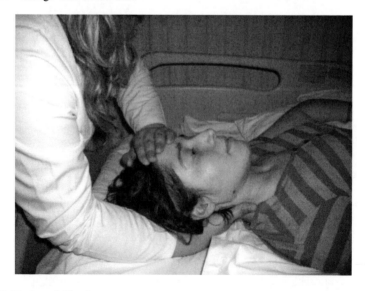

Figure 20. Neck mobilization.

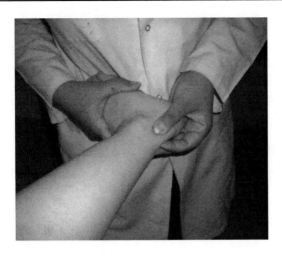

Figure 21. Ankle mobilization.

## 8.3.8. Vibration

Bishop has studied neurophysiological basis and therapeutic effects of vibration comprehensively [34]. Vibration should serve a single purpose for spastic patients, which can be defined as the inhibition of spastic muscle by facilitation of weak antagonist muscle through reciprocal inhibition.

Vibration generates a reflex contraction in the vibrated muscle by stimulating Ia fibers; this outcome is called tonic vibration reflex. Its effect is more extensive if vibration is applied directly on tendons [35]. In order to generate tonic vibration response, a high frequency vibration (100 to 300 hertz) should be applied. During the application, the muscle slowly and progressively increases its tone, reaching the peak point in 30 to 60 minutes; muscle tone is restored in plateau level throughout the stimulus. According to some researchers, a three-minute application is required for maximum tonic contraction. Holding the muscle in the most stretched position may be necessary to increase the effect of vibration. .

During vibration application, the points listed below should be considered:

- Vibration frequencies above 200 hertz may cause skin damage.
- The most ideal and secure frequency is 150 hertz.
- Patients with excessive sensory problems, such as disestesia and parestesia, should be exposed to vibration with utmost care and responses be observed closely.

When general literature is reviewed, studies analyzing the effects of vibration application on spasticity are quite few, and their findings are dissimilar. In one study made by Ahlborg et al., 14 patients with cerebral palsy were analyzed for eight weeks. Whole-body vibration was applied to 7 seven patients, and seven had resistance training. Consequently, vibration proved to moderate spasticity [36].

Jackson et al. studied acute effects of whole-body vibration on lower extremity muscle performance of MS patients. They cited that there was no significant alteration in peak torques of quadriceps and hamstring muscles following the application [37].

Methodological studies analyzing vibration reflex as a physiological response mainly consist of studies regarding whole-body vibration, which denotes the need for newer studies conducted on antagonist of the spastic muscle.


## 8.3.9. Electrical Stimulation

Muscle activation generated by Electrical Stimulation differs from voluntary muscle activation: In a voluntary muscle contraction, motor units fire asynchronously, with a larger proportion of type I, fatigue-resistant muscle fibers of the smaller motor units being recruited first. The order of muscle fiber firing occurs as a result of motor neuron size and the anatomy of synaptic connections. Conversely, an electrically stimulated muscle contraction elicits initial responses from larger motor units, which contain a greater number of fatigable, type II muscle fibers and motor units fire synchronously. A study of healthy subjects demonstrated recruitment of these higher threshold motor units at relatively low neuromuscular electrical stimulation training levels. This phenomenon is not possible with voluntary exercise, as much greater exercise intensity is required for activation of these larger motor units. In order to achieve beneficial outcomes, density of Electrical Stimulation, frequency of stimulus and resting periods should be considered along with patient profile.. However, there is no definite and reliable information on appropriate stimulation parameters, treatment duration and efficiency of the application [38].

Electrical Stimulation application on upper motor neuron lesions targets on strengthening the antagonist muscle and inhibiting spastic muscle. Electrical Stimulation used for these purposes has two forms of application: Neuromuscular Electrical Stimulation and Transcuteneal Electrical Nerve Stimulation (TENS). Neuromuscular Electrical Stimulation can be applied to the patient while resting or during function (Functional Electrical Stimulation (FES)).

Furthermore, studies regarding the moderation of spasticity through Electrical Stimulation are quite few in general literature. Functional Electrical Stimulation (FES) and Transcuteneal Electrical Nerve Stimulation (TENS) were employed in the above-mentioned studies.

FES is applied on antagonist of the spastic muscle during substantial functional movement. Antispastic effect is presumed to develop when spastic muscle is relaxed, resulting from reciprocal inhibition during the contraction in antagonist muscle [39]. Theoretically, strengthening of antagonist muscle in the long run should lead to an increase in the inhibitory effect of reciprocal inhibition on spastic muscle; and in addition, application of FES during the function might cause stimulation of spasticity in central nervous system. These are neural theories. When considered from a non-neural point of view, stimulation generates collateral blood vessels in the stimulated area and new capillaries develop. According to research, during a one-month period of Electrical Stimulation application programme, there was a 100% increase reported in capillary beds. When actin and myosin filaments within the muscle contract and contraction are transmitted to tendons, a sliding movement occurs. Following the sliding filament movement, physiologic range of motion exercise is applied. Activation of myosin flaments, proprioceptive input and cognitive sensory stimuli altogether decrease the intensity of spasticity, sustain the development of voluntary movement and result in the improvement of function [40].

According to some study reports, FES decreases spasticity; to some, it increases spasticity and to some, it does not affect spasticity at all [41]. Taylor et al. applied FES by using Odstock Dropped Foot Stimulator (ODFS) to fix dropped foot in patients with upper neuron lesions. Subjects belonging to different diagnostic groups participated in the study; each diagnostic group was then divided into two, regarding their prior experiences with the device: subjects who were introduced to the device recently and subjects who are already familiar with the device. One hundred twenty-three strokes, 18 MS, 10 SCI, five traumatic brain injuries and four cerebral palsy patients took a part in the study. Various questions regarding the usage of the device, effects of the device on their walk, spasticity and problems they encountered while using the device were asked to the subjects. Ninety-two subjects cited that ODFS was efficient on spasticity. According to 37% of these subjects, ODFS decreased spasticity, to 17.4% it increased spasticity and to 45.6%, the device did not affect spasticity [42].

Krause et al. reported that FES application decreased spasticity in lower extremity muscles of a single patient. FES was applied to gluteal muscle groups, quadriceps and biceps femoris muscle; then subject leg-cycled for 30 minutes. Spasticity was measured before and after two training sessions. Spastic muscle tone was measured clinically using MAS and semi automatically by pendulum testing of spasticity. Spasticity scores decreased following the exercise, and according to the subject, this effect lasted for several hours [43].

According to a study analyzing the effects of peroneal nerve stimulation on neuroprosthetics of MS, made by Sheffler et al., ODSF application resulted in an increase in ankle motion, improvement in balance and decrease in spasticity [44].

TENS selectively stimulates myosin proprioceptors of the skin and is usually used in the management of pain [45]. Its inhibitory effect mechanism on the muscle is not clear. The only explicate theory is about pain management. According to this theory, pain stimulates afferent reflex mechanisms and aggravates spasticity. Application of TENS reduces pain and moderates spasticity [1]. However, clinical experiences show that TENS application on the spastic muscle dermatome of patients having no pain complaints results in a decrease in muscle tonicity. Signals deriving from muscle fiber afferents are interfered by TENS application; this interference leads to an insignificant inhibition of stretch reflex, resulting in the moderation of spasticity. In literature, TENS is generally used to manage spasticity in neurological diseases; but there are only few studies concerning its application on patients.

Mattison applied TENS on MS patients while they were sleeping and observed a significant decrease in spasticity related to pain and sleeping disorders [46].

Armutlu et al. in their study analyzing MS, applied high-frequency TENS (*100 Hz and pulse width 0.3 msec*) to the corresponding dermatome, 20 min/day for four weeks in a group of patients with mild to moderate spasticity in the plantar flexor muscles of the ankle. Spasticity was assessed by using EMG, MAS and Ambulation Index. The results demonstrated a statistically significant reduction in spasticity according myoelectric activity and the MAS after four weeks of TENS application [47].

Miller et al. split 32 MS patients into two groups. For a period of two weeks, 60 minutes of TENS (100 Hz and 0.125 ms pulse width) per day was applied to the subjects in the first group, and eight hours of TENS per day was applied to the second group. Electrotes were placed on the quadriceps muscle and pulse intensity was increased to a degree that wouldn't lead to distress. Treatment was recessed for two weeks following the first session. Application duration was switched between the groups during the second session of the treatment. As a result, although TENS proved not to be efficient on moderating spasticity in particular, long-term applications were effective on pain management and muscle spasms [45].

As a consequence, TENS may be used to manage spasticity; however, its efficiency and success is determined by the effects of pain on a patient's spasticity. TENS may prove to be more effective on patients with spasticity that is increasing in conjunction with sensory stimulation and pain. More studies need to be conducted regarding the application of TENS on spasticities not accompanied with pain.

Besides these two methods, faradic or high voltage pulsed galvanic stimulation (HVPGS) may be used to strengthen antagonist muscle. Because of its tolerability, high voltage pulsed galvanic stimulation is more commonly preferred. This stimulation may be used either with pulses or with Russian technique: 20 seconds of resting after each ten seconds of stimulation for ten applications maximum (figure 22).

Cetişli et al. randomly split 33 patients into two groups. HVPGS was applied to antagonists of spastic muscles of the first group; repetitive contractions stimulated with PNF were applied to the second group. According to the findings of this four-week treatment, MAS scores of spastic gastro-soleus and quadriceps femoris muscle decreased more significantly in HVPGS group than PNF group. These findings show that Electrical Stimulation applied to antagonist of the spastic muscle activates reciprocal inhibition, thus strengthening the muscle and contributing to the relaxation of the spastic muscle [48].

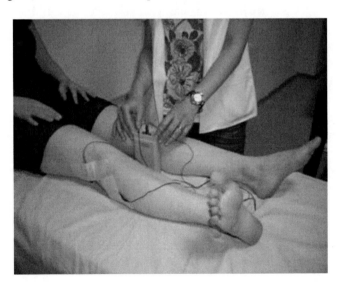

Figure 22. HVGS application to peroneal muscles.

## 8.3.10. Biofeedback

Biofeedback is applied to improve function during the acute and chronic phases of motor recovery. It is used to reduce improper contractions, to sustain weak antagonist muscle and to inhibit the spastic muscle. Biofeedback training is based on giving feedback to the patient about his personal performances via audio and visual stimulation. It can be applied in different formations. EMG biofeedback—in which superficial electrodes are used—is more commonly preferred. Biofeedback provides the patient with multimodal information. Audio signals may be used to maintain the proper head posture. Portable biofeedback devices can be used by patients personally when they are not under treatment to correct their posture, to manage unwanted movements during functions and to inhibit spastic muscle [35].

In a study aiming to determine the effects of EMG biofeedback on 59 patients by Lourenção et al., to 31 patients, the occupational therapy and FES accompanied by EMG biofeedback were applied twice a week. The remaining 28 patients were treated with occupational therapy and FES without EMG biofeedback. ROM, spasticity and hand functions of the patients were evaluated in the following two weeks, six months and 12 months. According to the six-month evaluation findings, all mentioned variables significantly improved statistically, and spasticity was moderated in the patients who had EMG biofeedback application [49].

## 8.3.11. Kinesiotape Application

Kinesiotape application has recently become popular. Kinesiotape has 140% elasticity matching that of the skin, giving non-restricted support that allows muscles to perform a full range of motion, easily and comfortably. Kinesiotaping gives support and stability to joints and muscles without affecting circulation and range of motion. The technique is based on the body's own natural healing process, exhibiting its efficacy through the activation of neurological and circulatory systems. Muscles are not only attributed to the movements of the body but also control the circulation of venous and lymph flows, body temperature, etc. Therefore, the failure of the muscles to function properly induces various kinds of symptoms.

Consequently, so much attention was given to the importance of muscle function that the idea of treating the muscles in order to activate the body's own healing process. By using an elastic tape, it was discovered that the muscles and the other tissues could be helped by outside assistance. Employment of kinesiotaping creates a totally new approach to treating nerves, muscles, and organs. The kinesiotaping method is applied over muscles to reduce pain and inflammation, relax over-used tired muscles, and support muscles in movement on a 24hr/day basis. It is non-restrictive type of taping that allows full range of motion.

According to a study conducted by Yasukawa et al. targeting children with neurological problems and spasticity, kinesiotape application increased the motor functions. Taping is assumed to support weak muscles and provide them with biomechanical advantages to generate movements and to contribute to sensory motor integration by procuring sensory feedback [50, 51]. This study emphasizes the theory that "improving the movement ability by supporting weak antagonist muscle results in a decrease in muscle tonicity through reciprocal inhibition" (figures 23 and 24).

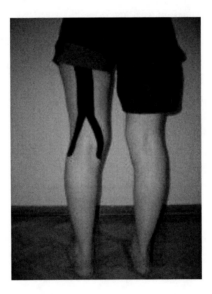

Figure 23. Kinesiotape application for weak hamstrings.

## 8.4. INDIRECT (GENERAL) APPROACHES

Indirect approaches are effective on hypertonic cases and neurophysiological problems. They provide a wide range of positive outcomes in physical therapy practice. The responses achieved through the use of indirect applications involve almost all body structures. They are used for the regulation of general body muscle tone and facilitation of voluntary movement patterns. Indirect approaches are categorized in two main groups, which are neuro-developmental methods and others.

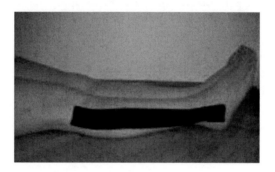

Figure 24. Kinesiotape application weak evertors.

## 8.4.1. Neuro-Developmental Treatment Methods

Neuro-developmental treatment methods were defined through the end of 1940s; acceptance of these methods and first publications took place in 1950s. With the development of these methods, physical therapy applications were freed from passive, limited and conventional techniques and became more effective. The basics of neuro-developmental treatment methods were established by Rood, Kabat and Knott, Brunnstrom and Bobath. In the following years, several alternative approaches and concepts were added, without the modification of basic principles. When literature is surveyed, it is observed that Bobath Concept is still the most popular of these methods. Therefore, the analysis of neuro-developmental treatment methods is hereby started with a review of Bobath Concept.

### Bobath Concept

According to Bobath, spasticity does not affect a single muscle but a large portion of the body; thus body posture and movement patterns are affected accordingly. Therefore, reflex inhibitory patterns and mat exercises are used to inhibit spasticity and manage tonic reflex activity (figures 25 and 26). Furthermore, the concept aims at sustaining coordination by generating normal activity reactions against abnormal movements and inhibiting abnormal patterns of the movement. Specific inhibition techniques, fixation and facilitation of balance reactions are used in order to actualize above-mentioned outcomes. Movement sense is used for the regulation of tone instead of stimulation of superficial sensory receptors (i.e., brushing, tapping, ice application, vibration). The physical therapist should follow the below mentioned steps in order to achieve inhibition and development of voluntary movement sense:

- In order not to stimulate stretch reflex, movements should be performed slowly; appropriate time should be reserved for inhibition between the movements.
- Spastic patterns should be inhibited via inhibition of antagonist patterns (reciprocal inhibition).
- For the inhibition of spastic patterns, the physiotherapist should apply placing; initial movements should be applied by the therapist to avoid increased muscle tone; patient participation should take place in the advanced stages. The physical therapist should stop the movement at the moment that he feels an increase in muscle tone and a low time for inhibition to occur.
- Facilitation and stabilization of voluntary movement should be actualized by the inhibition of hypertonus and the use of joint surface (with approximation).
- Patient should be taught to inhibit his spasticity by making use of specific movements (autoinhibiton). In Bobath approach, autoinhibitions are frequently used to control muscle tonicity.

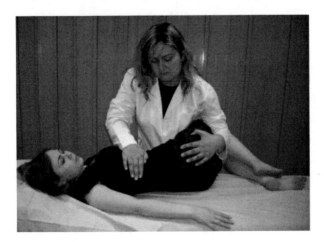

Figure 25. Trunk rotation and stretching of latissimus dorsi muscle.

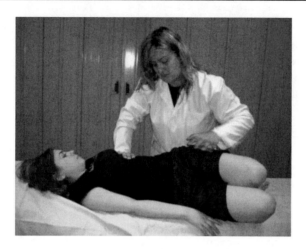

Figure 26. Trunk rotation and stretching of latissimus dorsi muscle.

In addition, periphery inputs, such as proprioceptive sense, may affect and alter motor outputs. Senses in proximal joints (shoulder, pelvis) and distal joints (wrist, ankle) are important in particular. These areas, called distal-proximal key points, should be positioned properly and correct sensory inputs should be delivered to generate correct movement in order to regulate muscle tonicity [52].

Although Bobath Concept is frequently used in clinical practice by physiotherapists working in the field of neurology, there is only one study on MS patients in general literature. The study, conducted by Smedal et al. on two MS patients, was focused more on balance deficits than MS, inquiring the effects of Bobath method on walking. Following the treatment period of two months, improvements on both parameters were observed [52].

Other studies are mostly conducted on stroke patients. A study conducted on ten patients with spasticity resulting from stroke analyzed the effects of Bobath approach on the excitability of spinal motor neurons. Plantar flexors of the patients were treated accordingly with Bobath approach, three times a week for ten sessions. Alfa motor activity before and after the treatment was evaluated by H reflex latency and Hmax/Hmax ratio. Also, ROM was determined and spasticity was measured with AS. Before the treatment, Hmax/Hmax ratio scores of ankle plantar flexors were higher than those of non-spastic ankle; however, H reflex latency and Hmax/Hmax ratio scores showed no signs of alteration after the treatment. In addition, Hmax/Hmax ratio scores of spastic ankle approximated the scores of normal ankle. According to AS findings, a significant decrease in spasticity and an increase in ankle ROM developed statistically [54].

A study carried out by Wang et al. on stroke patients with different motor levels compared Bobath approach with orthopedical approaches. Twenty-one of the 23 participant patients had different degrees of spasticity. In the study, Stroke Impairment Assessment Set, Motor Assessment Scale, Berg Balance Scale and Stroke Impact Scale were used to determine disorder and functional limitation levels. The muscle tonicity is measured with MAS. Subjects were treated according to Bobath approach and orthopedical approaches for four weeks and 20 sessions. Statistically, the intensity of spasticity decreased significantly in patients who were treated with Bobath approach [55].

### Johnstone Concept

This approach corresponds with normal developmental model and conversion is from proximal to distal. Firstly, the gross motor skills and secondly the fine motor skills are to be enhanced. Inhibition of abnormal pattern during the acute phase is fundamental. The approach aims at establishing a balance between the facilitory and inhibitory mechanisms of sensory motor neuromuscular system. In order to achieve this goal, pressure splints and positioning are used. Use of pressure splints differentiates Johnstone Approach from Bobath Approach. These splints are made from a transparent substance; they are manually inflated and are made up of several plates (arm, hand, leg, foot, etc) (figures 27, 28). Splints are applied to inhibit spasticity, manage associated reactions and generate necessary stabilization for extremity starting from an early stage. It is possible to explain the effect mechanism of pressure splints on inhibition of spasticity by their effects on autogenetic inhibition and their local regulatory role on the autonomic nervous system. Autogenetic inhibition is actualized by placing the splinter on antispastic position of extremity for 20 minutes. Local autonomic regulation is generated when neutral temperature created by lung air stimulates parasympathetic activity. Also, pressure applied by the splints result in a regular proprioceptive input [56].

There are no studies about the effects of Johnstone approach on MS spasticity in literature. One study conducted on MS patients made use of Jonhstone pressure splints, however, this study focused on ataxia [57]. This particular study was conducted by Kerem et al. regarding the effects of Johnstone splints on CP patients with spasticity. Bobath approach was applied on one group and Bobath method accompanied by Johnstone pressure splints was applied to the other group. As a consequence, it was seen that splint application had inhibitory effects on spasticity according to MAS [58].

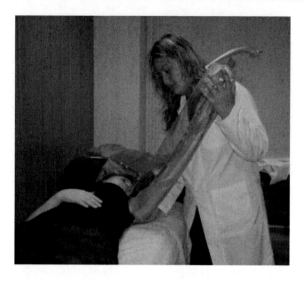

Figure 27. Pressure splint application for upper extremity.

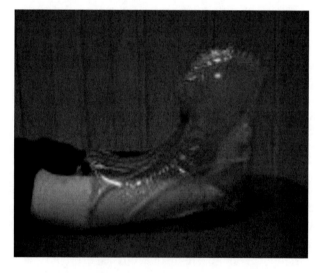

Figure 28. Pressure splint application for foot.

## *Rood Concept*

The basic approach of Rood method is the proper use of sensory stimuli, which employs all receptors and stimulation forms defined in the "Rood Chapter." The method aims at altering motor responses by applying appropriate sensory stimuli. Rood approach involves various tactile stimulants such as stroking, brushing, icing together with techniques like stretching and compression to inhibit spasticity. Brushing facilitates antagonist of spastic muscle. It implies the stimulation of nerve roots by using a soft brush or fingertips. Stimulation deriving from skin receptors increases fusimotor impulses of muscle fibers, enhancing the excitability of muscle fibers. There is no difference between stimulating the nerve root and stimulating the muscle or skin innervated; however, muscle and skin covering the muscle should be innervated by the exact same nerve root. Since muscle fiber stimulation develops slowly, brushing should be applied 20 minutes before the other treatment application and for just a few seconds on each area.

Another technique applied to facilitate antagonist muscle is icing. Ice cubes are rubbed rapidly and slightly on the muscle. Melted water should be prevented from dripping elsewhere. Icing is applied on muscles and skin innervated by the same nerve root.

Rood approach involves slow stretching to loosen the spastic muscle. This technique regulates the sensitivity of fibers towards tension in motor units of muscles with slow activation. The stretched muscle should not be biarticular. Stretching is applied at least for five minutes. Application of stretching on soleus muscle is performed in dorsiflexion direction when the knee is bended and leads to the stimulation of secondary endings on intrafusal muscle fibers in the deep fibers, resulting in facilitating the inhibitory antagonist of the relaxed muscle. Stretching may activate dorsiflexors that are antagonists of soleus inhibition, and facilitation of dorsiflexors may cause the inhibition of loosened antagonist muscles (gastrocnemius). Therefore, according to Rood, slow stretching is not an appropriate technique to be applied on biarticular muscles. (i.e.,gasrocnemius).

Another application of Rood technique to moderate extansory spasticity is stroking. Massage should be applied starting from the cervical area to caudal area rhythmically and slowly [32].

According to Rood concept, motor development of a movement has seven stages. Facilitation/inhibition achieved through sensory stimulation are used to enhance these stages. Rood also defined four stages to gain control over the movement. These stages are:

- Acquisition of total movement patterns.
- Development of postural stability.
- Acquisition of the ability to support the body by distal segments during movements.
- Restoration of normal patterns.

When literature is surveyed, it is seen that there are no studies regarding the Rood Concept.

## 8.4.2. Proprioceptive Neuromuscular Facilitation

Based on the principle that cerebrum manages movement not individually but in patterns, Knott and Kabat developed Proprioceptive Neuromuscular Facilitation (PNF) method, which emphasis diagonal patterns. In order to generate inhibition/facilitation within these patterns, PNF applies different techniques based on the neurophysiologic principles defined by Sherrington:

- *After discharge:* Stimulus effect continues after stimulation stops. If the strength and duration of the stimulus increase, the "after discharge" increases as well.
- *Temporal summation:* A succession of weak stimuli occurring within a certain period of time combines to cause excitation.
- *Spatial summation:* Weak stimuli applied simultaneously to different body parts reinforce one another to cause excitation. Temporal and spatial summation may combine for greater activity.
- *Irradiation:* This is spreading and increased strength of a response. It occurs when either the number or the strength of the stimuli is increased. The response may be either excitation or inhibition.
- *Successive induction:* An increased excitation of the agonist muscles follows stimulation of their antagonists. Techniques involving reversal of antagonists make use of this property.
- *Reciprocal innervation (reciprocal inhibition):* Contraction of muscles is accompanied by simultaneous inhibition of their antagonists. Reciprocal innervation is a fundamental part of coordinated motion. Relaxation techniques make use of this feature.

Facilitation of normal total movement pattern was assumed to sustain motor learning and secondarily to decrease spasticity and abnormal movement patterns. According to the PNF method, active muscle contractions are able to grow strong within the central nervous system via stimulation of afferent proprioceptive discharges, resulting in an increase in excitability and additional motor unites taking a part in the movement.

There are several sub techniques of PNF designed for alternative purposes, all maintaining neurophysiological basis. These can be listed as:

- Rhythmic Initiation
- Combination of Isotonics
  - o  Reversal of Antagonists
  - o  Dynamic Reversal of Antagonists
  - o  Stabilizing Reversal
- Rhythmic Stabilization
- Repeated Stretch
  - o  Repeated Stretch from beginning of range
  - o  Repeated Stretch through range
- Contract-Relax
- Hold-Relax
- Replication

Relaxation in the spastic muscle, on the other hand, may be actualized directly or indirectly by increasing the reciprocal inhibition of antagonist muscle via applications such as sudden stretching, strength expansion, resistance, etc. In the application of "contract-relax" (a direct application of PNF), spastic muscle is isometrically contracted against maximal resistance, the tension resulting from this contraction stimulates golgi tendon organ and loosens the spastic muscle by autogenetic inhibition [59, 60].

Following the inhibition of spastic muscle, rhythmic initiation and repeated stretch techniques are applied in order to strengthen weak antagonist muscle.

In general literature, there are no studies on the outcomes of PNF techniques on MS patients.

Etnyre and Abraham analyzed the effects of static stretch and contract-relax and contract-relax-antagonist-contract (a PNF technique) on the motor pool excitability of soleus muscle. Motor pool excitability was evaluated with H reflex. H-wave slightly decreased after the application of static stretching. PNF techniques proved to be far more efficient. Neural inhibitory might have contributional effects on decreasing motor pool excitability. Furthermore, a larger motor pool inhibition might decrease muscle contractibility, and thus, allow more muscle consistency. Consequently, PNF techniques, particularly the ones involving reciprocal activation, are more effective on muscle stretching [61].

### 8.4.3. Body Image and Sensory Integration Training

Body image disturbances in patients with upper motor lesions occur in forms of improper and stereotypical motor responses resulting from inadequate cortical organization of peripheric senses and senses deriving from deep body surface. Ayres defined these inadequacies and emphasized the necessity of sustaining perceptual motor functions in Acquisition patients with neurological damage. Although body image and sensory integration training is a part of physical therapy training, in practice, it is more commonly applied by occupational therapists. The training aims at sustaining sensory process by controlled sensory input and generating proper motor responses [62].

It should be kept in mind that MS patients, in particular, have intense sensory and perceptual problems, which may result in a disturbed body image; this, in return, will have negative effects on the severity of spasticity. A patient who is unable to understand his spatial position will not be able to perform a movement in the desired pattern, and while trying to do so, hypertonus may develop in different muscle groups. For instance, in the case of a patient who is unable to perform an upper extremity movement because he cannot relax his arm, he should be assisted by placing a pillow between his body and arm; this may help sustaining body image and reduce hypertonus.

### 8.4.4. Vestibular Stimulation

The vestibular apparatus is a mechanoreceptor. Peripheral proprioceptive receptors inform the CNS where the body is in space, and the vestibular system relays information about the head position and linear acceleration in space. Because the vestibular system is intimately connected to the visual, proprioceptive, and motor systems, it works interactively to modulate important functions. The vestibular system has been credited with influencing muscle tone and maintaining visual gaze, spatial directionality, and clarity of the image when the head or an object is moving, and head and body orientation.

Beneficial outcomes gained by stimulation of a system having such significant functions through specific inputs should be considered and used as a reinforcing factor for the physiotherapy programmes. Because any static position as well as any movement pattern will facilitate the labyrinthine system, vestibular function plays a role in all therapeutic activities. To conceptualize vestibular stimulation as spinning or angular acceleration minimizes its therapeutic potential and also negates an entire progression of vestibular treatment techniques.

Horizontal, vertical, and forward-backward movements occur very early in development and should be considered one viable treatment modality. A constant, slow, repetitive rocking pattern, irrespective of plan or direction, generally causes inhibition of total-body responses, whereas a fast spin or fast linear movement tends to heighten both alertness and the motor responses [63].

Since vestibular stimulation generates its effects by facilitating/inhibiting the connections between vestibular system and brainstem, Ayres used this stimulation in sensory integration trainings [35].

When subjects with spasticity are seated on a rocking chair or hammock and swung with a speed of less than 30 km/per minute, vestibular path is inhibited. This leads to a decrease in ventral horn activity of the body and extremity extensors, resulting in relaxation [35].

Slow vestibular stimulation is employed to actualize inhibition. Slow repetitive swinging or rotational movements may be applied as active-assistives or passive. By using a rocking chair, therapy ball, pillow, balance board or wheelchair, sitting, rotating and tumbling exercises can be performed. Furthermore, vestibular stimulation may be applied in combination with orthosis (PAFO or pressure splints), respiratory exercises and relaxation techniques in a quiet environment [64] (figure 29).

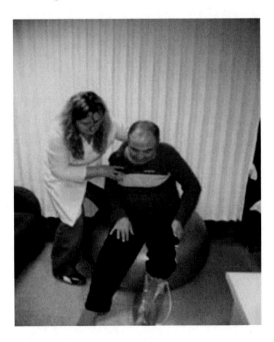

Figure 29. Vestibular stimulation on the therapy ball.

Occasionally, vestibular stimulation application may have side effects (i.e., nausea, vertigo, dizziness, etc.) in patients with sensitive vestibular system. In such cases, the physical therapist should apply alternative methods.

## 8.4.5. Hippotherapy

Hippotherapy stimulates the patient's normal reactions. The goal of hippotherapy is to stimulate locomotion, improve the balance and coordination of movement, normalize muscle tension, and eliminate pathological reflexes [65]. Hippotherapy may affect balance, gait, spasticity, functional strength, coordination, pain, self-rated level of muscle tension, activities of daily living and health-related quality of life [66].

During therapeutic horse-riding, the hip adductors remain fixed in an antispastic position for a long duration, enabling autogenetic inhibition; parasympathetic system is stimulated by the neutral body heat of the horse, causing a relaxation in the whole body, and the vestibular system is stimulated by rhythmic movements, resulting in a temporary inhibition of spasticity. The rhythmic back-and-forth movement of the pelvis generates an expanded rhythmic movement in a key area of the body, leading to a general relaxation throughout the body.

When the literature is reviewed, it is seen there are two studies analyzing the effects of hippotherapy on MS patients. One of the studies questions the effects of hippotherapy on postural control. The other is carried out by Hammer et al. Eleven MS patients were applied hippotherapy for ten weeks and symptoms such as postural control, lower extremity spasticity and pain were evaluated. Consequently, measured by MAS, a statistically significant decrease in lower extremity spasticity was reported [66].

Studies regarding hippotherapy are focused mostly on patients with cerebral palsy and spinal cord injuries. The findings of these studies show that therapeutic horse-riding moderates spasticity for a short period of time [67, 68].

## 8.4.6. Hydrotherapy

Hydrotherapy is one of the oldest methods applied for the management of physical dysfunctions. It is used for warming or cooling body segments, muscle relaxation, overcoming joint limitations and psychological relaxation.

Giesecke defines the goals of aquatic exercises as moderating spasticity, increasing peripheral circulation, sustaining aerobic endurance and psychological efficacy [69].

Including hydrotherapy in the treatment designed to moderate spasticity may contribute to the success of the programme. Since MS patients are heat intolerant, water temperature should be set up between 27 to 29 °C during the hydrotherapy session. This heat is the equivalent of normal temperature. Hydrotherapy may be more efficient if the patients perform aquatic exercises. Inhibition of spastic muscles may be explained with the effects of neutral temperature on autonomic nervous system and with the increase in proprioceptive inputs generated by the pressure applied by water. The difference of aquatic exercises from those performed on land is that body temperature does not increase during aquatic exercises. The stabilization of body temperature minimalizes pseudo exacerbations—including spasticity—of MS symptoms [19]. In addition, by supporting impaired muscles, water itself may ease the exercises and help to strengthen muscles.

Hydrotherapy is usually applied in forms of free-swimming in the pool (to sustain aerobic capacity), walking in the water (to strengthen weak antagonist muscles) and stretching. In addition, techniques such as Badragaz and Halliwick may also be applied to strengthen the weak muscles. The most important thing in hydrotherapy application is to make sure that the water is hygienic.

## 8.4.7. Reflexology

The effect of reflexology on MS symptoms is recently defined. The method involves applying pressure on parts of the feet with thumb or finger. It is based on the theory that internal organs, glands and other body segments are mirrored on the feet [70]. Its difference from foot massage is that reflexology involves deep-pressure massage—defined as caterpillar-like movements—application to reflex areas. It is asserted that pressure applied on reflex zones block energy, spread elements such as calcium, lactate, etc., and reabsorb disposed uric acid crystals. Reflexology is also assumed to reset homeostasis by reducing tension and stress and increasing the flow of blood to particular body segments. It is presumed to be an efficient method in pain reduction, healing of wounds and improving the quality of sleep. Also physical contact is believed to be beneficial for the patient's psychological health [71].

In a study conducted by Siev-Nerl et al. on the effects of reflexology on MS patients, 71 subjects were split into two groups. Reflexology involving foot and calf massage was applied to the experimental group for 11 weeks. On the other hand, only calf massage was applied to the control group. Muscle strength, urinary symptoms, paresthesia and spasticity of the patients were evaluated before, immediately after 1.5 and three months of the treatment. Spasticity was measured with AS. In the experimental group, a significant decrease in paresthesia, urinary symptoms and spasticity was observed [72].

## 8.5. CONCLUSION

MS is a complex disease in terms of symptoms and treatment applications. Spasticity, which is a major symptom of the disease and a crucial factor aggrevating the severity of disabilities, is more complex than MS itself. Management of spasticity demands a multidisciplinary approach. Minimal spasticity is manageable by using physiotherapy merely, whereas treatment of moderate and severe spasticity may involve myorelaxant medication, botilinum toxin application and surgical operations. In such cases, interdisciplinary communication and consensus should be maintained, goals and application of treatments should carefully be determined. For instance, high-dose myorelaxan medication may have negative effects on a patient with ataxia and muscle impairment in conjunction with spasticity. His muscle tonicity may decrease while his disability is increasing. Therefore, medication dosage should be determined both by a neurologist and a physiotherapist working together. In cases with local spasticity, combining physical therapy with botox injection proves to be an efficient treatment. Botox injection, which is quite an expensive treatment, is not efficient alone; therefore, strengthening exercises should immediately be applied following the injection.

A number of physiotherapy techniques developed to decrease spasticity are reviewed in this chapter, stressing mainly the factors such as "the choice of treatment techniques by the clinician, under different conditions," is always the consequential and crucial question. The localization (muscles, number of muscles and functions affected by spasticity), the time elapsed following the occurrence of spasticity, muscle stiffness, joint limitations and sensory loss should be taken into consideration by an experienced physiotherapist for the determination of an appropriate and valid method.

During the preparation of this chapter, it was seen that there was a large number of physiotherapy techniques and surveys focusing on the moderation of spasticity available in literature, whereas the studies and techniques concerning

MS patients were few and limited in number. Hopefully, future conduction of more studies regarding the effects of physiotherapy applications on MS patients with spasticity will arouse interest in the subject and contribute to further developments of new techniques.

## 8.6. REFERENCES

[1]   Watanabe, T. (2004). The Role of therapy in spasticity management. *Am J Phys Med Rehabil,* 83 (suppl), S45–S49.

[2]   Lee, S.U. & Bang, M.S.& Han, T.R. (2002) Effect of cold air therapy in relieving spasticity: applied to spinalized rabbits. *Spinal Cord,* 40(4),167-73.

[3]   Price, R. & Lehmann, J.F. (1990). Influence of muscle cooling on the viscoelastic response of the human ankle to sinusoidal displacements. *Arch Phys Med Rehabil,* 71(10), 745-748.

[4]   Bell, K. R. & Lehmann, J. F.(1987). Effect of cooling on H and T-reflexes in normal subjects. *Arch of Phys Med Rehabil,* 68, 490-3

[5]   Lehmann, J. F. & deLateur, B. J. (1982) Cryotherapy. In Lehman J.F. (eds.), *Therapeutic Heat and Cold,* (editon 3, pp: 563-602). Baltimore: Williams & Wilkins.

[6]   Chiara, T. & Carlos, J. & Martin, D. & Miller R. & Nadeau S. (1998). Cold effect on oxygen uptake, perceived exertion, and spasticity in patients with multiple sclerosis. *Arch Phys Med Rehabil,* 79, 523-528.

[7]   Petrilli, S. & Durufle, A. & Nicolas, B. et al. (2004) Influence of temperature changes on clinical symptoms in multiple sclerosis: an epidemiologic study. *Ann Readapt Med Phys,* 47, 204–208.

[8]   Nilsagård, Y. & Denison, E. & Gunnarsson, L.G. (2006). Evaluation of a single session with cooling garment for persons with multiple sclerosis—a randomized trial. *Disabil Rehabil Assist Technol.* 1(4), 225-33.

[9]   Neurological Rehabilitation. Umphred DA (ed). Umphred D, Byl N, Lazaro R. Interventions for Neurological Disabilities chapter 4, (4. Edition). Mosby company, St. Louis, 2001.

[10]  Schmit, B.D. & Dewald, J.P. & Rymer, W.Z. (2000). Stretch reflex adaptation in elbow flexors during repeated passive movements in unilateral brain-injured patients. *Arch Phys Med Rehabil,* 81(3), 269-78.

[11] Vattanasilp, W. & Ada, L. & Crosbie, J. (2000). Contribution of thixotropy, spasticity, and contracture to ankle stiffness after stroke. *J Neurol Neurosurg Psychiatry,* 69(1), 34-9.

[12] Nuyens, G.E. & De Weerdt, W. & Ketelaer, P. & Spaepen, A. & Staes, F. (2001). Torque variations during repeated passive isokinetic knee movements in persons with multiple sclerosis. *J Rehabil Med,* 33 (2), 85-9.

[13] Nuyens, G.E. & De Weerdt, W.J. & Spaepen A.J. & Kiekens, C & Feys, H.M. (2002). Reduction of spastic hypertonia during repeated passive knee movements in stroke patients. *Arch Phys Med Rehabil,* 83(7), 930-5.

[14] Bovend'Eerdt, T.J. & Newman, M. & Barker, K. & Dawes, H. & Mineli, C. & Wade D.T. (2008). The effects of stretching in spasticity: a systematic review. *Arch Phys Med Rehabil,* 89, 1395-406.

[15] Brar, S.P. & Smith, M.B. & Nelson L.M. & Franklin G.M. & Cobble N.D. (1991). Evaluation of treatment protocols on minimal to moderate spasticity in multiple sclerosis. *Arch Phys Med Rehabil.* 72(3), 186-189.

[16] Giovannelli M, Borriello G, Castri P, Prosperini L, Pozzilli C. Early physiotherapy after injection of botulinum toxin increases the beneficial effects on spasticity in patients with multiple sclerosis. *Clin Rehabil,* 2007 Apr;21(4):331-7.

[17] Yeh, C.Y. & Chen, J.J. & Tsai, K.H. (2004). Quantitative analysis of ankle hypertonia after prolonged stretch in subjects with stroke. *J Neurosci Methods,* .30; 137(2),305-14.

[18] Yeh, C.Y. &, Tsai, K.H. & Chen, J.J. (2005). Effects of prolonged muscle stretching with constant torque or constant angle on hypertonic calf muscles. *Arch Phys Med Rehabil,* 86(2), 235-41.

[19] White, L.J. & Dressendorfer, R.H. (2004). Exercise and multiple sclerosis. *Sports Med,* 34(15), 1077-100.

[20] Buttler, D.S. (1989). Adverse mechanical tension in the nervous system: a model for assessment and treatment. *Aust J Physiother,* 35:227-238.

[21] Buttler, D.S. (1991). *Mobilization of the Nervous System,* New York, Churchill Livingstone.

[22] Ellis, R.F. & Hing, W.A. (2008). Neural mobilization: a systematic review of randomized controlled trials with an analysis of therapeutic efficacy. *J Man Manip Ther,* 16(1), 8-22.

[23] Saunders, D.G. & Walker, J.R. & Levine, D. (2005). Joint mobilization. *Vet Clin North Am Small Anim Pract,* 35(6):1287-316.

[24] Maricar, N & Shacklady, C. & McLoughlin L. (2009). Effect of Maitland mobilization and exercises for the treatment of shoulder adhesive capsulitis: a single-case design. *Physiother Theory Pract,* 25(3):203-17.

[25]  Edward, S. (1996). *Neurological physiotherapy: a problem-solving approach.* (edition 1). New York: Churchill Livingstone.

[26]  Nash, B. & Roller, J.M. & Parker, M.G. (2008) The effects of tone-reducing orthotics on walking of an individual after incomplete spinal cord injury. *J Neurol Phys Ther*, 32(1), 39-47.

[27]  Pizzi, A. & Carlucci, G. & Falsini, C. & Verdesca, S. & Grippo, A. (2005). Application of a volar static splint in post stroke spasticity of the upper limb. *Arch Phys Med Rehabil*, 86, 1855-9.

[28]  Hazneci, B. & Tan, A.K.& Guncikan, M.N. & Dincer, K. & Kalyon, T.A. (2006). Comparison of the efficacies of botulinum toxin A and Johnstone pressure splints against hip adductor spasticity among patients with cerebral palsy: a randomized trial. *Mil Med*, 171(7), 653-6.

[29]  Lannin, N.A. & Herbert, R.D. (2003). Is hand splinting effective for adults following stroke? A systematic review and methodologic critique of published research. *Clin Rehabil*, 17(8), 807-16.

[30]  Fleuren, J.F. & Nederhand, M.J. & Hermens, H.J. (2006). Influence of posture and muscle length on stretch reflex activity in post-stroke patients with spasticity. *Arch Phys Med Rehabil*, 87(7), 981-8.

[31]  Wyke, B. D. (1972). Articular neurology. A review. *Physiotherapy*, 53(3), 94-99.

[32]  Banks, A. M. (1986). *International Perspectives in Physical Therapy 2: Stroke* (edition 1). Broadway, New York: Churchill Livingstone.

[33]  Venturini C, Penedo MM, Peixoto GH, Chagas MH, Ferreira ML, de Resende MA. Study of the force applied during anteroposterior articular mobilization of the talus and its effect on the dorsiflexion range of motion. *J Manipulative Physiol Ther*, 2007 Oct;30(8):593-7.

[34]  Bishop B. Vibratory stimulation: II. Vibratory stimulation as an evaluation tool. *Phys Ther*, 55:29-33,1975.

[35]  Gelber, A. & Douglas, R.F. (2002). *Clinical evaluation and management of spasticity* (1 edition). Totowa, New Jersey: Humana Press.

[36]  Ahlborg, L. & Andersson, C. & Julin, P. (2006). Whole-body vibration training compared with resistance training: effect on spasticity, muscle strength and motor Performance in adults with cerebral palsy. *J Rehabil Med*, 38, 302-308.

[37]  Jackson, K.J. & Merriman, H.L. & Vanderburgh, P.M. & Brahler, C.J. (2008). Acute effects of whole-body vibration on lower extremity muscle performance in persons with multiple sclerosis. *J Neurol Phys Ther*, 32(4), 171-6.

[38] Nelson, C. & Hacke, J.D. & Mcculloch, K.L. Electrodiagnosis and Electrotherapeutic Intervention. In Umphred, D.A. (editor). *Neurological Rehabilitation*, (4. Edition). Mosby company, St. Louis. (2001).

[39] Thompson, A.J. & Jarrett, L. & Lockley, L. & Marsden, J. & Stevenson, V.L. (2005). Clinical management of spasticity. *J Neurol Neurosurg Psychiatry*, 76, 459-463

[40] Weingarden, H.P. & Zeilig, G. & Heruti, R. & Shernesh, Y. & Ohry, a. & Dar, A. & Katz, D. & Nathan, R. & Smith, A. (1998). Hybrid functional electrical stimulation orthosis system for the upper limb: Effects on Spasticity in Chronic stable Hemiplegia. *Am J Physic Med & Rehabil*, 77 (4) : 276-281.

[41] Sköld, C. & Lönn, L. & Harms-Ringdahl, K. & Hultling, C. & Levi, R. & Nash, M. & Seiger, A. (2002). Effects of functional electrical stimulation training for six months on body composition and spasticity in motorcomplete tetraplegic spinal cord-injured individuals. *J Rehabil Med*, 34, 25–32.

[42] Taylor, P. N. & Burridge, J.H. & Dunkerley, A.L. & Lamb, A. & Wood, D.E. & Norton, J.A. & Swain, I.D. (1999) Patients' perceptions of the Odstock Dropped Foot Stimulator (ODFS). *Clin Rehabil, 13;* 439-446.

[43] Krause, P. & Szecsi, J. & Straube, A. (2007). FES cycling reduces spastic muscle tone in a patient with multiple sclerosis. *Neuro Rehabilitation*, 22, 335–337.

[44] Sheffler, L.R. & Hennessey, M.T. & Knutson, J.S. & Chae, J. (2009). Neuroprosthetic Effect of Peroneal Nerve Stimulation in Multiple Sclerosis: A Preliminary Study. *Arch Phys Med Rehabil*, 90,362-365.

[45] Miller, L. & Mattison, P. & Paul, L. & Wood, L. (2007). The effects of transcutaneous electrical nerve stimulation (TENS) on spasticity in multiple sclerosis *Multiple Sclerosis*, 13, 527-533.

[46] Mattison, P. (1993). Transcutaneous electrical nerve stimulation in the management of painful muscle spasm in patients with multiple sclerosis. *Clin Rehabil*, 7, 45-48.

[47] Armutlu, K. & Meriç, A.& Kırdı, N. & Yakut, E. & Karabudak, R. (2003). The effect of transcutaneous electrical nerve stimulation on spasticity in multiple sclerosis patients: a pilot study. *Neurorehabil Neural Repair*, 17, 79-82.

[48] Çetişli, K.N. & Kırdı, N. & Armutlu, K. & Keser, İ. & Karabudak, R. (2007). Improvement in multiple sclerosis patients' spasticity obtained with high voltage pulsed galvanic stimulation. *Multiple Sclerosis Clinical and Laboratory Research*, Vol 13, Suppl. 2, poster 446.

[49] Lourenção, M.I. & Battistella, L.R. & de Brito, C.M. & Tsukimoto, G.R. & Miyazaki, M.H. (2008). Effect of biofeedback accompanying occupational therapy and functional electrical stimulation in hemiplegic patients. *Int J Rehabil Res,* 31(1), 33-41.

[50] Simoneau, G. & Degner, R. & Kramper, C. & Kittleson, K. (1997). Changes in ankle joint proprioception resulting from strips of athletic tape applied over skin. *Journal of Athletic Training,* 32, 141–147.

[51] Murray, H. & Husk, L. (2001). Effect of kinesio taping on proprioception in the ankle. *J Orthopedic Sports Physical Therapy,* 31, A-37.

[52] Bobath, B. (1990). *Adult Hemiplegia: Evaluation and Treatment* (3rd Edition). London: Heinemann.

[53] Smedal, T. & Lygren, H. & Myhr, K.M. & Moe-Nilssen, R. & Gjelsvik, B. & Gjelsvik, O. & Strand, L.I. (2006). Balance and gait improved in patients with MS after physiotherapy based on the Bobath concept. *Physiother Res Int,* Jun;11(2):104-16.

[54] Ansari, N.N. & Naghdi, S. (2007). The effect of Bobath approach on the excitability of the spinal alpha motor neurones in stroke patients with muscle spasticity. *Electromyogr Clin Neurophysiol,* 47(1), 29-36.

[55] Wang, R.Y. & Chen, H.I. & Chen, C.Y. & Yang, Y.R. (2005). Efficacy of Bobath versus orthopedic approach on impairment and function at different motor recovery stages after stroke: a randomized controlled study. *Clin Rehabil,* 19(2), 155-64.

[56] Johnstone, M. (1987). *Stroke patient: A team approach.* (3rd Edition). Edinburg: Churchill Livingstone.

[57] Armutlu, K. & Karabudak, R. & Nurlu, G. (2001). Physiotherapy approaches in the treatment of ataxic multiple sclerosis: a pilot study. *Neurorehabil Neural Repair,* 15(3):203-11.

[58] Kerem, M &, Livanelioglu, A. & Topcu, M. (2001). Effects of Johnstone pressure splints combined with neurodevelopmental therapy on spasticity and cutaneous sensory inputs in spastic cerebral palsy. *Dev Med Child Neurol,* May;43(5):307-13.

[59] Kabat, H. Proprioceptive Neuromuscular Facilitation in Therapeutic Exercise, (In) Licht, S. (Ed), *Therapeutic Exercise* (edition 2, p.p:327-343), Baltimore, Maryland: Wavverly Press.

[60] Knott, M. & Voss, D.E. (1968). *Proprioceptive Neuromuscular Facilitation.* (2nd edition). New York, Harper and Row Publishers.

[61] Etnyre, B.R. & Abraham, L.D. (1986). H-reflex changes during static stretching and two variations of proprioceptive neuromuscular facilitation techniques. *Electroencephalogr Clin Neurophysiol,* 63(2), 174-9.

[62] Mateer, C. (1997). Rehabilitation of individuals with frontal lobe impairment, in Neuropsychological Rehabilitation: Fundamentals, Innovations, and Directions (Leon Carrington, J. ed), St. Lucie Press, Delray Beach, FL.

[63] Farber S: A multisensory approach to neurorehabilitation. In Farber S (ed): Neurorehabilitation : A multisensory approach, Philadelphia, WB Saunders, 1982.

[64] Dreeben, O. (2007). *Physical Therapy Clinical Handbook for PTAs.* Boston: Jones and Bartlett Publisher.

[65] Lisiński, P. & Stryła, W. (2001). The utilization of hippotherapy as auxiliary treatment in the rehabilitation of children with cerebral palsy. *Ortop Traumatol Rehabil,* 3(4), 538-40.

[66] Hammer, A. & Nilsagård, Y. & Forsberg, A. & Pepa, H. & Skargren, E. & Oberg B. (2005). Evaluation of therapeutic riding (Sweden)/hippotherapy (United States). A single-subject experimental design study replicated in eleven patients with multiple sclerosis. *Physiother Theory Pract,* 21(1), 51-77.

[67] Lechner, H.E. & Kakebeeke, T.H. & Hegemann, D. & Baumberger, M. (2007). The effect of hippotherapy on spasticity and on mental well-being of persons with spinal cord injury. *Arch Phys Med Rehabil,* 88(10), 1241-8.

[68] Lechner, H.E. & Feldhaus, S. & Gudmundsen, L. & Hegemann, D. & Michel, D. & Zäch, G.A. & Knecht, H. (2003). The short-term effect of hippotheraph on spasticity in patients with spinal cord injury. *Spinal Cord,* 41(9), 502-505.

[69] Giesecke C. Aquatic rehabilitation of clients with spinal cord injury. (1997). In: Ruoti, R.G. & Morris, D.M. & Cole, A.J.(eds). *Aquatic rehabilitation* (edition 1, pp:125-150). Hagerstown: Lippincott, Williams and Wilkins.

[70] Botting D. (1997) Review of literature on the effectiveness of reflexology. *Complementary Therapies in Nursing & Midwifery,* 3, 123-130.

[71] Wang, M.Y. & Tsaı, P.S. & Lee, P.H. & Chang, W.Y. & Yang, C.M. (2008) The efficacy of reflexology: systematic review. *J Advanced Nursing,* 62(5), 512–520.

[72] Siev-Ner, I. & Gamus, D. & Lerner-Geva L. & Achiron A. (2003). Refiexology treatment relieves symptoms of multiple sclerosis: a randomized controlled study. *Multiple Sclerosis,* 9, 356-361.

In: Spasticity and Its Management ...
Editor: Kadriye Armutlu

ISBN: 978-1-60876-185-5
© 2010 Nova Science Publishers, Inc.

*Chapter 9*

# RELAXATION AND ENERGY CONVERSATION TECHNIQUES

## *Ayla Fil and Yeliz Özçelik*

Hacettepe University, Faculty of Health Sciences, Department of Physical
Therapy and Rehabilitation, Neurological Rehabilitation Unit,
06100/Ankara/TURKEY

## 9.1. ABSTRACT

Relaxation is total physical relaxation of the skeletal muscles with a regulatory effect on the sympathetic nervous system. Even while resting, muscles are never completely relaxed; they maintain a specific tone. When muscle tone increases, it results some negative effects such as rapid heartbeat and cold hands. Relaxation techniques like Respiratory Exercise and Progressive Relaxation Technique can eliminate these effects. Increasing stress and muscle tone can cause loss of energy. Fatigue is a very important problem in MS. It limits patients in their lives. In addition to this, spasticity and fatigue affect each other. So Energy Conservation Techniques are used to prevent fatigue and to increase muscle tone.

Key words: relaxation, fatigue, energy conservation.

## 9.2. INTRODUCTION

Relaxation may be described as a state in which there is total physical relaxation of the skeletal muscles with a regulatory effect on the sympathetic nervous system. This is accompanied by a feeling of diminished consciousness of the external world, passivity and focusing of the attention on feelings of internal well-being.

Even while resting, muscles are never completely relaxed; they maintain a specific tone. However, some emotional factors such as anger cause further increase of muscle tonicity. Increased muscle tone results in a rapid heartbeat, respiration frequency and coldness in feet and hands. Relaxation techniques are designed to eliminate these negative effects caused by stress. A relaxed person is able to breathe deeply and easily, his hands and feet are warm, he has a calm heartbeat and his muscles are relaxed, indicating slowed body metabolism.

Relaxation exercises have quite positive outcomes on patients suffering from MS, headache, asthma and cardiac diseases. Including relaxation exercises in treatment programmes of diseases like MS, in which spasticity, painful cramps, fatigue and autonomic dysfuntions are commonly observed, will enable the patient to benefit more from physiotherapy. However, it should be kept in mind that relaxation exercise does not function as a treatment method when applied individually; it helps the patient to perform other exercises more efficiently with a minimum effort.

## 9.3. RELAXATION TECHNIQUES

In order to actualize relaxation, the patient should wear comfortable clothes that are not tight and the environment should be dim and tranquil. The head of the patient should be supported by a pillow and semiflexion should be maintained by placing a pillow under the knees; this will avert the distress caused by shortened hamstrings as well. Occasionally, respiratory exercises may be required for the achievement of complete relaxation. Slow and controlled respiration should be maintained throughout the relaxation exercises in progress.

### 9.3.1. Example of Respiratory Exercise

Respiratory exercises should be controlled by the mind, applied slowly, deeply and quietly. The physical therapist should give the below-listed instructions to the patient in a low and smooth tone of voice:

- Close your eyes and focus only on the movements of your abdomen. Concentrate on your breath while your abdomen moves upwards with inhalation and downwards with exhalation.
- Take a deep breath with your nose and feel the fresh air filling your lungs. Exhale from your mouth as slowly as possible.
- During respiratory exercises, sentences enhancing concentration may be used, such as "when I inhale, my lungs are filled with cold, fresh air and as I exhale hot and filthy air slowly comes out of my lungs. I feel calm and refreshed."
- Relaxation exercises should involve approximately five to ten minutes of respiratory exercises, until a controlled respiration is achieved. This period of respiratory exercise varies from one patient to another because of the individual differences.

### 9.3.2. Progressive Relaxation Technique

The technique, developed by Jacobson in 1920s, is based on the contraction and relaxation of major muscle groups [1]. Thereby, the difference between tension and relaxation is clearly felt by the patient.

During the progressive relaxation technique, the patient sits or lies down thoroughly supported. He is asked to inhale and exhale slowly, eyes closed. The patient is instructed as: "lift your left wrist, hold it up for one minute, release it for three minutes, and repeat this order twice. Try to perceive the difference between contraction and relaxation." The same contract-release order should be repeated for the right hand, arms, legs, neck, body and the area surrounding the eyes.

### 9.3.3. Accelerated Progressive Relaxation Technique

The technique was developed by Bernstein and Borkovec in 1973. It is based on the same philosophy as Jacobson's. During the exercises, five to ten seconds of contraction and 30 to 40 seconds of relaxation is practiced. Below are the instructions:

- Clasp your hands, contract your forearm and release.
- Clasp your dominant hand; pull your wrist towards the chair. Repeat the order with your other arm.
- Raise your eyebrows, crinkle your nose, clench your teeth, push your chin backwards.
- Force your head backwards.
- Push your shoulder backwards.
- Contract your abdominal muscles.
- While bending your knee, push your ankle downwards; while straightening your knee, pull your ankle upwards. Repeat the same order with your other leg [2].

### 9.3.4. Biofeedback

The technique, defined by Basmajian and De Luca in 1985, eased the acquisition of relaxation by the patient under instruction. During biofeedback, patient's physiological reactions such as body temperature, perspiration, heartbeat and blood pressure are conveyed to the patient himself by using audio and visual signals. Thereby, the patient becomes aware of the alterations within his own body and tries to keep them under control. However, not the whole body but only some specific muscle groups can be relaxed with the use of this method. It should be practiced along with other techniques to achieve complete relaxation [3].

### 9.3.5. Autogenetic Relaxation Technique

Autogenetic relaxation technique was developed by Schultz and Luthe. It is practiced in sitting or lying down position of the patient and involves the use of relaxing visual demonstrations. The technique focuses on six responses of a relaxed body [4].

- Weight
- Warmth
- Cardiac adjustments

- Respiration
- Warmth of abdomen
- Stiffness of the forehead

Aside from these techniques, alternative methods such as reciprocal physiological relaxation, yoga and meditation may be exercised to achieve relaxation.

## 9.4. ENERGY CONSERVATION TECHNIQUES

Fatigue is one of the major MS symptoms that has negative effects on the daily life of the patient. MS fatigue is different from that of healthy people [5].

Pathophysiology and etiology of fatigue is not clarified at present; however, it is assumed that both peripheral and central mechanisms have a part in the development of fatigue [6, 7].

Spasticity, in particular, pain, nocturia, sleep disorders and body temperature regulation defects, are factors aggravating MS fatigue.

Treatment of MS fatigue requires a multidisciplinary approach. The patient should be informed about medicative treatment (for moderation of fatigue), exercise treatment, management of spasticity, behavioral modification and energy conservation techniques.

Energy conservation and reduction of workload is based on the awareness of specific factors that may be the causes of various cardiovascular responses. Ogden has defined six variables increasing the need for oxygen, which can be listed as: rapid heartbeat, increased resistance, increased usage of major muscle groups, increased usage of trunk muscles, raising the arms and isometric activities. Upper extremity activities require more cardiovascular output than activities of lower extremity, i.e., standing requires more energy than sitting. Heat, humidity and polluted air cause the over-activity of the heart.

Considering the above-mentioned principles, MS patients may be advised to:

- Perform working activities in sitting position.
- Organize working area by preparing the required equipments beforehand.
- Eliminate unnecessary activities and combine required activities.
- Avoid lifting heavy objects or use equipment to lift and carry loads (avoid bending down).
- Use electrical devices when possible.

- Arrange materials in a way that gravity will be of assistance for completing the movement.
- Arrange the required activity in a specific order and give time off to rest for days/weeks.
- Let other people do some of the work.
- Make daily or weekly programmes and split chores that require extra energy.

Numerous studies have been conducted regarding energy conservation techniques and the moderation of MS fatigue [8, 9, 10].

Most of the studies are based on the energy conservation method developed by Packer et al. Packer et al. instructed their patients in a six-week course programme for energy conservation [11].

| Sessions | Content of session |
|---|---|
| Session 1: The Importance of Rest | Basic Terminology and Concepts: Fatigue, fatigue in MS, gradual passive change<br>Energy Management: Banking and budgeting energy, working on a balance<br>Practice Activity/Homework: Finding time to rest, creating a rest schedule |
| Session 2: Communication and Body Mechanics | Homework Review: Difficulties and successes<br>Communication: Attitudes of others, hidden disability, communicating your needs<br>Banking: Don't Waste Energy/Use good body mechanics:<br>Postures, lifting, & carrying<br>Practice Activity/Homework: Communication and body mechanics |
| Session 3: Activity Stations | Homework Review: Difficulties and successes<br>Banking: Don't Waste Energy: Apply ergonomic principles to work stations, use energy-efficient tools at home and |

| | at work<br>Practice Activity/Homework:<br>Designing and rearranging an activity<br>station |
|---|---|
| Session 4: Priorities and Standards | Homework Review: Difficulties and successes<br>**Banking: Don't Waste Energy:** Activity analysis and modification<br>Budgeting Energy: Evaluation of priorities and standards for daily activities<br>Practice Activity/Homework: Priorities and standards, planning a day |
| Session 5: Balancing Your Schedule | Homework Review: Difficulties and successes<br>Living a Balanced Life: Taking control: Analyzing and modifying a day<br>Practice Activity/Homework: Actual vs. real day, planning a week |
| Session 6: Course Review and Future Plans | Homework Review: Difficulties and successes<br>Review of Course Content: Energy management/banking and budgeting energy<br>Practice Activity: Short- and long-term goal setting<br>Feedback and Course Evaluation |

In a study by Sauter et al., 32 MS patients were included in a course for energy conservation, for six weeks and two hours a day. The course was translated from German to English and underwent several cultural adaptations. Fatigue Severity Scale, the MS-specific Fatigue Scale, the Modified Fatigue Impact Scale (MFIS), the Pittsburgh Sleep Quality Index, a self-rating scale for depression, The Expanded Disability Status Score (EDSS) and the MS Functional Composite (MSFC) scores of patients were assessed before and after the course programme; assessments were repeated following the seventh and ninth months. Significant statistic alterations were observed in MFIS total score and cognitive and physical sub score of patients in both follow-up assessments, whereas no such alteration was observed in scores of fatigue Severity Scale, MS-specific Fatigue Scale and Psychosocial Fatigue Impact Scale. After the week course programme, MSFC and EDSS scores of patients remained the same as pre-course. Sleep quality of patients showed improvement, and their depression scores were decreased in the post-course and during the next seven- to nine-month assessments [8].

In another study regarding the effects of six-week energy conservation course on fatigue, quality of life and self-efficacy was carried out by Mathiowetz et al. on 169 randomized MS patients. The findings were assessed by using Fatigue Impact Scale (FIS), quality of life SF-36 Health Survey and Self-Efficacy for Performing Energy. As a consequence, when compared with the control group, FIS subgroup of treatment group had a significant decrease in physical and social scores statistically and an increase in Vitality sub scale of SF-36. In addition, Conservation Strategies Assessment increased significantly post course compared to pre-course [10].

## 9.5. CONCLUSION

In MS patients, local spasticity is frequently accompanied by agitation and alertness resulting from sympathetic over activation (developed primarily with the disease). Due to spasticity and stiffness in muscles, a patient may encounter muscular fatigue in addition to disease-related fatigue. In such excessive fatigue cases, the physiotherapist may apply relaxation techniques to patient, as a pre- and post-treatment programme. Beneficial outcomes of relaxation and physical therapy exercises are enhanced if supported by the application of energy conservation techniques, which minimalizes fatigue and moderates spasticity, aggravated due to the effort spent during exercises.

## 9.6. REFERENCES

[1] Jacobson, E. (1938). *Progressive relaxation.* Chicago: University of Chicago Press.
[2] Bernstein, D. A. & Borkovec, T. (1973). *Progressive relaxation: A manual for the helping professions.* Champaign, Research Press.
[3] Basmajiani J.V. & DeLuca, C.J. (1985). *Muscle alive: their functions revealed by electromyography.* (5th Ed.) Baltimore: Williams & Wilkins.

[4]     Luthe, W. & Schultz, J.H. *Autogenic Therapy*, (first published) by Grune and Stratton, Inc., New York, (1969). Republished in (2001) by The British Autogenic Society.

[5]     Djaldetti, R. & Ziv, I, Achiron, A. & Melamed, E. (1996). Fatigue in multiple sclerosiscompared with chronic fatigue syndrome: A quantitative assessment. *Neurology,* 46:632-635.

[6]     Tartaglia, M.C. & Narayanan, S. & Francis, S.J. & Santos, A.C. & De Stefano, N. & Lapierre, Y. & Arnold, D.L. (2004). The relationship between diffuse axonal damage and fatigue in multiple sclerosis. *Arch Neurol,* 61:201-207

[7]     Bakshi, R. (2003). Fatigue associated with multiple sclerosis: diagnosis, impact and management. *Mult Scler,* 9:219-227.

[8]     Sauter, C. & Zebenholzer, K. & Hisakawa, J. & Zeitlhofer, J. & Vass, K. (2008). A longitudinal study on effects of a six-week course for energy conservation for multiple sclerosis patients *Multiple Sclerosis*, 14: 500–505.

[9]     Finlayson, M. (2005). Pilot study of an energy conservation education program delivered by telephone conference call to people with multiple sclerosis. *Neuro Rehabilitation*, 20: 267–77.

[10]    Mathiowetz, V.G. & Finlayson, M.L. & Matuska, K.M. & Chen, H.Y. & Luo, P. (2005). Randomized controlled trial of an energy conservation course for persons with multiple sclerosis. *Mult Scler*, 11: 592–601.

[11]    Packer, T. L. & Brink, N. & Sauriol, A. (1995). *Managing fatigue: A six-week course for energy conservation.* Tucson, Arizona: Therapy Skill Builders.

In: Spasticity and Its Management …
Editor: Kadriye Armutlu

ISBN: 978-1-60876-185-5
© 2010 Nova Science Publishers, Inc.

*Chapter 10*

# CASE HISTORY: PROBLEM SOLVING

### *Kadriye Armutlu**

Hacettepe University, Faculty of Health Sciences, Department of Physical
Therapy and Rehabilitation, Neurological Rehabilitation Unit
06100 /Ankara /TURKEY

## 10.1 INTRODUCTION

Physical therapy and rehabilitation is a long and difficult process targeting on patient oriented functional improvement and social participation. In chronic and progressive diseases like MS, this process requires cooperative efforts of the patient, his relatives, caretakers, rehabilitation team, and the physical therapist in particular.

Throughout the rehabilitation process, most frequently visited member of the team by MS patient is the physiotherapist. Due to progressive character of MS, physical therapist may encounter different findings and problems during each visit. Applications concerning the altered condition of the patient should be assessed immediately. Physical therapist should have a good knowledge about the causes of patient's problems and be able to develop programmes concerning these new outcomes. His approach is expected to be flexible and problem-solving based.

Problem-solving is a learned ability improved by therapist's individual clinical experiences and theoretical knowledge. During problem-solving, steps listed below should be followed:

* Email: karmutlu@hacettepe.edu.tr

Taking a good case history and close observation of the patient

Main problem obstructing daily life activities of the patient should be inquired

Functional improvement expectations of the patient from treatment should be noted

Basic problem of the patient and possible alternative problems leading to it should be schematized.

A treatment method for each problem should be determined.

This chapter involves a case history in order to provide the reader with information on spasticity-related problem solving.

# 10.2. CASE

Male patient, 44 years old, married, has a child, an architect. Applies to the clinic to receive physical therapy treatment for the first time since his MS had been diagnosed.

**Story**: He consulted a neurologist with a complaint of random double–vision 8 years ago. According to examination results and analysis, he was diagnosed MS. Following his visit, pulse-steroid was applied intravenously for 5 days and his complaint of double vision diminished.

Subsequently, he felt a slight heaviness and lack of control on his left leg. His neurologist decided on the prolonged application of intravenous pulse- streoid treatment once again but this time medication did not generate dramatic effects. After two years, pulse-steroid application was discontinued and immunosupresan treatment was initialized, by use of immuran. In the last 4 years new complaints such as contraction and stiffness in left calf muscles, loss of strength in left leg and falling down resulting from his toe brushing the ground, have developed. He used tizanidine for the moderation of spasticity for some time but discontined because the medication was deficient in moderating contractions and stiffness and had side-effects (slight sedation and xerostomia). He had no attacks during these 8 years.

The patient is presently diagnosed with progressive MS and medicated with immuran and L-Carnitine.

**Patient's present clinical picture**: slight left hemiparesis on the lower extremity,

*Complaints*: He has difficulties and needs support while ascending/descending stairs and slopes; stiffness in left calf muscles, minimal disability in left hand

*Anticipated functional gain attained from physical therapy*: ability to ascend / descend stairs and slopes easily, without support.

*Assessments*: observational gait analysis has been conducted on the patient in order to determine factors obstructing the patient while ascending / descending stairs and slopes.

According to the findings of walking analysis; the factors generating postural instability during stair and slope climbing activity are:

Insufficient knee control during standing phase (hyperextension)

Insufficient ankle movement during push-off

Foot limited in plantar flexion position results in excessive hip flexion while trying to pull foot off the ground

Weakness of dorsiflexor caused by gastronecmius spasticity and limitation of ankle joint on plantarflexion position lead to further difficulties in keeping knee joint under control (knee hyperextention).

**Other assessment parameters:**
- ✓ EDSS score
- ✓ Proprioception of knee joint (passive motion sense)
- ✓ Two point discrimination sense of sole
- ✓ Joint motions of ankle joint (goniometric measurements)
- ✓ Hypertonicity (Modified Ashworth Scale)
- ✓ Increased tonic response to rapid movement and clasp knife phenomenon (neural / non-neural component)
- ✓ Manuel muscle testing
- ✓ Posture analysis
- ✓ Single limb stance duration (second)
- ✓ Berg Balance Scale
- ✓ Questioning of fatigue

Treatment programme was planned in consideration of assessment findings and patient's expectations. It involved stages listed below:

➢ **Direct approaches**
- Non-neural component of patient's spasticity was evident, therefore deep soft tissue mobilization (deep function massage) was applied on gastrosoleus. During the application, patient was in lying prone position and his ankle was fixed in maximal dorsiflexion. Prior to

soft tissue mobilization, cold pack was applied to ankle joint for 20 minutes, to minimalize pain.

- After joint mobilization was applied to ankle in order to overcome dorsiflexion limitations.
- Shrinked and tense tissues of foot sole were relaxed by use of 3 minute soft tissue massage; followed by deep frixion massage application to enhance the proprioceptive sense.
- Following joint and soft-tissue mobilization; 5 minute prolonged stretching to ankle was applied in two positions: while knee was in straight flexion (for gastronecmius) and in 90 ° flexion position (for soleus)
- Electrical stimulation (HVPGS and Russian technique), initialized with 5 repeats and finalized with 10 repeats in the advanced stages of the treatment was applied to strengthen weakened tibialis anterior and evertor muscles.
- Subsequently, these two muscles were strengthened by using PNF repeated stretch technique.

> **Indirect approaches and others**
- PNF repeated stretch technique was applied lying face-down position due to loss of strength in hamstrings. In the advanced stages of treatment, strengthening exercises of hamstrings was applied in standing position with supports accompanied by PNF combination of isotonics technique.
- Knee control was activated in lying down position and foot supported in dorsiflexion, in order to moderate loss of control in knee resulting from weakness, strength instability and decreased proprioceptors in m. quadriceps femoris and hamstrings.
- Abduction adduction control in bridge position was applied to strengthen weakened gluteus maximus and gluteus medius muscles and develop stabilization of pelvis.
- Closed kinetic chain exercises was applied to strengthen left gluteus medius (climbing the step with right leg while standing on left extremity)
- Multi-angular isometric quadriceps femoris training (holding each position for 1 minute) was practiced in order to enhance strength of quadriceps femoris in different angles.

At the end of 3 months treatment programme, patient was able to actualize knee control almost normally in short walks and static standing position. However, during long distance walks, knee angle control vanished and foot tip was again rubbing the ground. Therefore a mutual decision was made by the physical therapist and patient to use orthosis. Posterior leaf PAFO with 3 ° dorsiflexion was applied to patient, however patient was not comfortable with the application (sweating complaint), so it was discontinued.

Whereupon, kinesiotape application was practiced in order to support weak muscles and improve awareness. Kinesiotape was applied accordingly to support hamstrings and tibialis evertors and tibialis anterior.

By the end of the 4th month, patient developed knee control and postural control; his ability to ascend / descend stairs and slopes, improved.

Starting from the first day, the treatment programme was accompanied by home exercises. Patient is still being monitorized by follow-up examinations every 3 months and his well-being is steady.

**Home Exercises**
- Deep self-massaging on calf and foot sole
- Self-stretching of ankle
- Active-assistive dorsiflexion and eversion exercises
- Controlled knee flexion  (with support) in lying face-down and standing position
- Abduction adduction control in bridge position

- Bending right activity in sitting position

- Multi-angular isometric quadriceps femoris training while leaning against the wall (stay for 1 minutes in each position)
- Rolling a ball under foot by using different knee angles in lying down or sitting position

- Pressurizing the ball with left foot while standing on right foot position

- Rising on left toes deriving support from hands

- Walking training with mini-squats

**Needs support while ascending/descending stairs and slopes**

**CAUSES**

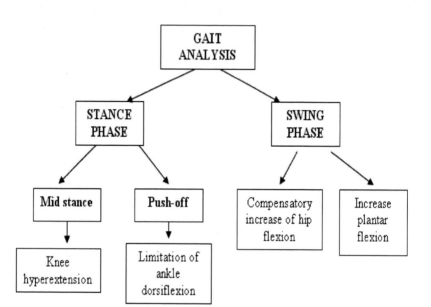

Analysis of the contribution of ankle joint to this circle:

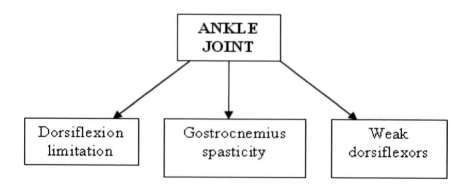

# 10.3. RESULTS

## TREATMENT 1

| | Pre-treatment | | Post-treatment | |
|---|---|---|---|---|
| 1-Angle of knee joint in mid stance phase | Right: 5° flexion<br>Left: -5° flexion | | The same | |
| 2-Proprioception of knee joint | Left knee flexion<br>80 70<br>30 40<br>60 50 | Righ knee flexion<br>80 78<br>30 25<br>60 60 | Left knee flexion<br>80 65<br>30 40<br>60 40 | Right Knee Flexion<br>80 70<br>30 20<br>60 50 |
| 3-Two point discrimination sense of sole | Left sole<br>Fore of sole: 2.5 cm<br>cm    fore of sole 3 | Right sole<br>Fore of sole: 1.5 cm<br>Back of sole: 2 cm | Left sole<br>Fore of sole: 3 cm<br>Back of sole : 3.5 cm | Right sole<br>Fore of sole: 2cm<br>Back of sole : 2.5 cm |
| 4-Joint motion (goniometric measurement) | Left ankle DF<br>Active limitation: 55°<br>Passive limitation: 48° | Right ankle DF<br>Active limitation: 20°<br>Passive limitation: - | Left ankle DF<br>Active limitation: 50°<br>Passive limitation: 40° | Right ankle DF<br>Active limitation: 20° |
| 5-Hipertonicity (MAS) | Left gastrosoleus mucle: 1+(undependent from speed) | | The same | |
| 6-Manuel mucle testing | | Left         Right | | |
| | Iliopusuas | 3+         5 | | |
| | Gluteus maximus | 3         5 | | |
| | Gluteus medius | 3         5 | | |
| | Internal rotators | 3         5 | The same | |
| | Quadriceps femoris | 3+         5 | | |
| | Hamstrings | 3         5 | | |
| | Gastrosoleus | 3         5 | | |
| | Tibialis anterior | 2         5 | | |
| | Perenoels | 2         5 | | |
| | Tibialis posterior | 4         5 | | |
| | Extensor hallucis longus | 4         5 | | |
| | Lateral abdominals | 3         4 | | |
| 7- Single limb stance duration (second) | Left : 4 second<br>Right : 60 second | | Left : 6 second<br>Right : 60 second | |

EDSS: 3.5

Posture: Modarate anterior balance

Berg Balance Scale score: 50

Fatigue: -

# TREATMENT 15

| | Pre-treatment | Post-treatment |
|---|---|---|
| 1- Angle of knee joint in mid stance phase | Right: 5° flexion: Left: -3° flexion | Left : -3° |
| 2- Proprioception of knee joint | Left knee flexion 80 75 / 30 39 / 60 52; Right knee flexion 80 78 / 30 25 / 60 60 | Left knee flexion 80 70 / 30 40 / 60 45; Right Knee Flexion 80 70 / 30 20 / 60 50 |
| 3- Two point discrimination sense of sole | Left sole Fore of sole: 1.5; fore of sole 2; Right sole Fore of sole: 1,5 / Back of sole: 2 | Left sole Fore of sole: 2,5 / Back of sole : 2,5; Right sole Fore of sole: 2 / Back of sole : 2.5 |
| 4- Joint motion ( goniometric measurement) | Left ankle DF Active limitation: 20° Passive limitation: 35°; Right ankle DF Active limitation: 15° Passive limitation: - | Left ankle DF Active limitation: 20° Passive limitation: 30° |
| 5- ipertonicity (MAS) | Left gastrosoleus mucle: 1 (undependent from speed) | 1 ( but its more soft) |

## 6- Manuel mucle testing

| Muscle | Left | Right | Post-treatment |
|---|---|---|---|
| Iliopusuas | 4 | 5 | |
| Gluteus maximus | 3 | 5 | |
| Gluteus medius | 3 | 5 | |
| Internal rotators | 3+ | 5 | |
| Quadriceps femoris | 3+ | 5 | |
| Hamstrings | 3 | 5 | |
| Gastrosoleus | 3+ | 5 | 3˙ |
| Tibialis anterior | 3 | 5 | 3˙ |
| Peroneals | 3 | 5 | |
| Tibialis posterior | 4 | 5 | |
| Extensor hallucis longus | 4 | 5 | |
| Lateral abdominals | 3+ | 4 | |

| | Pre-treatment | Post-treatment |
|---|---|---|
| 7- Single limb stance duration (second) | Left : 18 second Right: 60 second | Left : 20 second Right :60 second |

EDSS: 3.5

Posture: Slight anterior balance

Berg Balance Scale score: 53

Fatigue: -

Analysis of the contribution of knee joint to this circle:

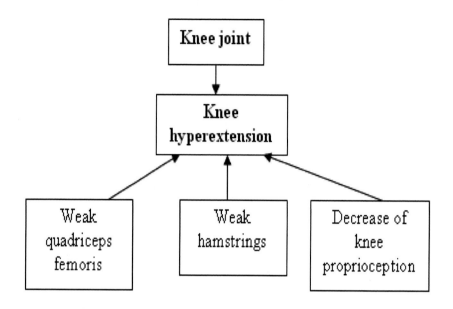

## 10.4. CONCLUSION

Above reviewed case is important in terms of proving that management of spasticity can be actualized by physical therapy applications. The case had minimal spasticity; however, his spasticity was chronic resulting in development of alterations in intrinsic muscle structure and ankle contraction. Using his problem-solving skills, physiotherapist determined the main problem of patient through observation and analysis and applied a complementary treatment accordingly. Consequently, both patient and therapist fulfilled their goals. What should be kept in mind is that, frequent and close follow-up examination of MS patients is important for the continuity of beneficial outcomes and management of newly-developed problems.

# INDEX

## D

## J

## K

## L

## T